10/2017

Communities of
Health Care Justice

Critical Issues in Health and Medicine

Edited by Rima D. Apple, University of Wisconsin–Madison, and Janet Golden, Rutgers University, Camden

Growing criticism of the U.S. health care system is coming from consumers, politicians, the media, activists, and healthcare professionals. Critical Issues in Health and Medicine is a collection of books that explores these contemporary dilemmas from a variety of perspectives, among them political, legal, historical, sociological, and comparative, and with attention to crucial dimensions such as race, gender, ethnicity, sexuality, and culture.

For a list of titles in the series, see the last page of the book.

Communities of Health Care Justice

Charlene Galarneau

Rutgers University Press

New Brunswick, New Jersey, and London

Library of Congress Cataloging-in-Publication Data
Names: Galarneau, Charlene, author.
Title: Communities of health care justice / Charlene Galarneau.
Other titles: Critical issues in health and medicine.
Description: New Brunswick, New Jersey : Rutgers University Press, [2016] | Series: Critical
issues in health and medicine | Includes bibliographical references and index.
Identifiers: LCCN 2016008284| ISBN 9780813577678 (hardcover : alk. paper) | ISBN
9780813577661 (pbk. : alk. paper) | ISBN 9780813577685 (e-book (epub)) | ISBN
9780813577692 (e-book (web pdf))
Subjects: | MESH: Community Health Services—ethics | Social Justice—ethics | Health
Policy | Socioeconomic Factors | United States
Classification: LCC RA399.A3 | NLM WA 546 AA1 | DDC 362.10973—dc23
LC record available at http://lccn.loc.gov/2016008284

A British Cataloging-in-Publication record for this book is available from the British
Library.

Visit our website: http://rutgerspress.rutgers.edu

Manufactured in the United States of America

Contents

Acknowledgments

I am grateful beyond words to the many who helped make this book possible. A 2012–2013 research leave from Wellesley College gave me the essential ingredient of time for this project, and the College's generous faculty research and conference travel grants are much appreciated. The Women's and Gender Studies Department has given me a lively academic home that has been unfailingly supportive of my research, and for this I thank Rosanna Hertz, Susan Reverby, Elena Tajima Creef, Irene Mata, Nancy Marshall, Jennifer Musto, Betty Tiro, Dulce Natividad, Sima Shakhsari, and Tanya McNeill. Special thanks go to Rosanna Hertz for facilitating my relationship with Rutgers University Press. Wellesley student research assistants extraordinaire Kayla Scire, Jane Adkins, and Elizabeth (Lily) Stowell provided valuable and engaged research assistance. Mark Schlesinger has been an abiding mentor and conversation partner since my graduate school days, for which I am profoundly grateful. Irene Mata and Tanya McNeill of the "Mighty Writers" group and Charlotte Harrison gifted me with their substantial and critical feedback, which has saved me from some silly and some substantial mistakes. At Rutgers University Press I thank Senior Editor Peter Mickulas, who paved the road to publishing with humor and responsiveness; Janet Golden and Rima D. Apple, editors of the Critical Issues in Health and Medicine Series that this book now joins; and two anonymous reviewers. Friends and family helped me keep mind, body, heart, and soul nourished with research breaks involving delicious food, walks in the woods, and surprise visits, as well as with tenacious support through this intensely solo and heady work—for this, my great appreciation goes to Sandy McCarthy, Rebekah Miles, Suzanne Seger, Jane Katz, John Field, and my sisters, Michele Gregg and Lisa Galarneau-Belisle. The late Frances Kornbluth, whose art graces the cover of this book, was a wise friend who urged me to just get this writing done. Dorothy and Paul Grout deserve special recognition and thanks, for they have created and shared a beautiful place apart in Vermont that has sustained me and my writing over the last near decade. My deepest gratitude goes to my partner, Don Tucker, who has always encouraged my work, read every word, and who opportunely trained for and ran two marathons while I wrote this book.

Communities of Health Care Justice

Introduction

This book expands the familiar ethical claim that health care is a social good, typically understood to mean that health care is a societal or national good. But "social" is a multilayered term, and *Communities of Health Care Justice* centers on the underappreciated notion that health care is also a community good, with community at this point meaning diverse groups typically smaller than society and larger than most families—groups internally connected by culture, religion, locale, or illness, for example. To say that health care is a community good is to say that social relations at the community level are essential to health care. If health care is, at least in part, a community good, then *just* health care must involve communities as well as the nation and individuals.

This project began with my effort to locate communities in some prominent theories of justice for health care and then to discern the moral work that these communities do in relation to justice. I found that, on the whole, these theories pay little attention to communities and that attention tends to frame communities as either morally irrelevant or morally problematic in relation to justice. In an attempt to recognize the diverse roles that communities play in health and health care and to position communities as critical moral participants in *just* health care, I present the notion of community justice, rooted in a principle of respect for all persons in their communities and involving three ethical norms: inclusive geographic communities, whole-person care, and participation as effective voice. Moreover, I show how these essential norms or criteria are located in contemporary U.S. health policy, albeit in limited ways. Notably this project takes me in the opposite direction of the current conceptual trend of scaling up national paradigms of justice for health care to the global level. Instead, I focus on subnational communities in order to address more fully the social relations—that is, the community relations—that I believe are most central to just health care.

Communities are morally important in just health care because, among many reasons, much U.S. health care (the context for this book) is done by communities in communities and for communities and because "we" do not care well for persons "we" consider to be outside "our" communities—witness the treatment of undocumented persons and uninsured persons. Inadequate health care puts lives at risk, and persons who are at risk of having relatively unhealthy and shortened lives are typically members of the same groups: They are members of low-income communities and communities of color. But this is not a book about inequities in health status or access to health care in the usual sense. It is about inequities in participation in the creation of just health care. Community justice is about putting in place standards of community, care, and participation that enable inclusive and respectful community involvement in health care. Community justice recognizes that different communities have different levels of power and privilege and that these inequities make a moral difference. Ultimately community justice has roots in the value of respect for persons and their communities, for virtually all persons are community members in ways that are important to their health and health care. As Heather Widdows and Sean Cordell point out, "Respecting individuals requires respecting communities and their goods, for it is individuals who suffer if the public and communal goods of their communities are not recognized and respected."[1]

I learned early in life how intertwined sickness, health care, and communities are. My father was seriously ill with Type I diabetes and its complications for more than five years before he died at age thirty-two. When he could no longer work, my mother got a job as a billing clerk in the local community hospital where my father would be a patient for weeks, even months, at a time. My mother's employment meant we had private health insurance. And the hospital once wrote off an unpaid bill amounting to hundreds of dollars, an act that earned my mother's loyalty throughout her work at, and retirement from, that same hospital thirty-four years later. Our small town—particularly our immediate neighbors, the elementary school my sisters and I attended, and Saint Catherine's, the Catholic community of working-class families of French Canadian descent, of which we were members—supported us in countless needed ways during those years.

My point is that we were part of the local health care community, and belonging to it and other communities meant that we were cared for in critical ways. In hindsight, I am certain that our being white, cis-gendered, U.S. citizens and my parents being a married, heterosexual couple privileged us in ways not accorded to all persons. As becomes clear in this book, the inclusion of all persons in health care communities is one requisite element of community justice.

My early work experiences in Colorado with community and migrant health centers in rural, low-income, mixed white and Latin@ communities, and then with a statewide association of like health centers, taught me more about communities, health, and justice. I understood well that health and health care were unevenly distributed across and within different communities. And

I believed that more and better health care providers were the answer: more community-based health centers that responded to community needs and more culturally competent health care workers motivated by a sense of social justice. I knew that poverty; discrimination by race, ethnicity, gender, and immigration status; poor housing, food, and education; and more played a big part in making people sick. But I persisted in focusing on health care as the primary means to change. Eventually I came to believe that these clinics would always have a long line out the door, so to speak, because they were embedded in a larger, and unjust, health care system—and society—that made it difficult, if not impossible, to adequately meet the health care needs of these communities.

Now, years later, I better understand the systemic and structural dimensions of health care and justice, with one such dimension being communities. Communities are central to how people understand and value health and health care. Communities contribute significantly to human health. Communities are home to many of the interpersonal and institutional caring relations that constitute health care. And communities benefit importantly from health care, as do individuals. While nations and families, too, embody social relations important to health care, the focus of this book is how these community dimensions relate to justice in U.S. health care.

Starting Points and Assumptions

Why do I address health care when, generally speaking, the social determinants of health have such a great influence on health status and when public health, with its population orientation, appears more conducive to community-level analyses? Health care, to my mind, is one aspect of public health, one determinant of health, and a disproportionately significant one for those communities and groups that experience disproportionate disease and injury. Moreover, the dominance of health care in the context of health creation calls for its critical moral examination.

The term "community" has been and continues to be the subject of extensive scrutiny, especially when used to describe an ostensibly homogeneous, harmonious, and inclusive social group.[2] And, as Emilie Townes contends, "Community can be a concrete site of strength and meaning making for engaged citizens."[3] Persons are deeply social and relational beings, and communities are among the many layers of relationality within which we live our lives. We identify with and participate in diverse communities to varying degrees across time and place. Complicated as they are, communities shape our health and our health care and cannot be ignored or simply disparaged.

"It is doubtful that [justice] can be made in only one way," says Michael Walzer, and this statement is affirmed by the abundance of theories of justice: justice as distributive, procedural, and participatory as well as institutional, structural, interpersonal, and more.[4] Justice is also multidimensional in part owing to the multidimensional forms of injustice. Justice, says Iris Marion Young, requires listening: "While everyday discourse about justice certainly makes claims, these are not theorems to be demonstrated in a self-enclosed system. They are instead calls, pleas, claims *upon* some people by others. Rational reflection on justice begins in a hearing, in heeding a call, rather than in asserting and mastering a state of affairs, however ideal. The call to 'be just' is always situated in concrete social and political practices that precede and exceed the philosopher."[5] Justice in health care, too, requires a hearing and a heeding, starting with respectful consideration of the calls and claims made by communities within the concrete social and political realities of the United States. As such, this book does not offer a specific national policy prescription, though community justice certainly has implications for national and community health policy.

Chapter Overviews

Chapter 1 develops the claim that health care is a community good and asserts the foundational relevance of communities and community relations for justice in health care. I attend to the nature of community and the definition of community used here before settling into the chapter's central focus: an elaboration of four significant community dimensions of health and health care—in other words, four ways that communities are critically associated with health and health care in the United States today: (1) Communities are significant sites of meaning making, that is, they are groups within which we create and re-create our understandings and values regarding health and health care. (2) Communities, especially local communities, provide physical and social environments that importantly affect our health. (3) Health care itself is an expression of caring relations at the community level. (4) Finally, communities benefit from health care in multiple ways that exceed individual health improvement.

Having established the import of communities and their relations to health care, and thus arguably their import to justice in health care, in chapter 2 I examine a range of the foremost liberal theories of justice in health care for their treatment of communities. On the whole, these theories pay little attention to communities, but when communities are addressed, they are acknowledged as religious or cultural communities or as communities united by race, class, or gender. These two clusters of communities tend to be treated differently: The religious or cultural communities are typically portrayed as obstacles or threats to justice, while race/gender/class communities are represented as disadvantaged victims and morally inert in relation to justice in health care. While still searching for a just health care theory that recognizes communities and their values as morally central to just health care, in chapter 3 I assess the liberal communitarian vision articulated by Ezekiel Emanuel. This framework, while promising in its high regard for community-based conceptions of the good life as essential to just health care, is limited by its narrow scope of justice, its rather distorted representation of communities as homogeneous and radically independent, and its inattention to the need for new mechanisms for meaningful community participation in decision making.

Offering a community-centered concept of justice in health care, in chapter 4 I present community justice—a vision that ultimately rests on the moral principle of respect for persons understood as inclusive of respect for communities. An institutional sketch of what U.S. health care characterized by community justice *might* look like provides systemic context for my principal contribution: the moral account of community justice. This moral vision of community justice consists of three ethical norms: that the health care community is inclusive and geographic; that health care cares for whole persons, both sick and well; and that participation in health care requires the effective voices of the multiple and diverse communities that make up the larger health care community. Together these three norms establish standards of justice that govern the health care activities of communities.

On the one hand, this vision of community justice seems far from current health care arrangements. On the other hand, given the multiple and varied notions of justice embedded in U.S. health care, elements of community justice (or approximations thereof) are found in contemporary health policy. In chapter 5 I locate various expressions—from glimpses to clear views—of community justice in three "moments" in U.S. health care: community health centers, the community health needs assessments that are required of nonprofit hospitals, and community-based health advocacy groups. From community-member-governed boards of health centers to the voices enabled by the organizing of activist advocacy groups, elements of community justice exist in health policy in small and large ways today. Finally, in the conclusion I integrate these justice moments and point to prospects for greater community justice.

Chapter 1

Health Care as a Community Good

We are still trying to define health as a social good. And this is good. It is a return of the practices of health to the people in the sense of governing health by the meanings we share.

—Jon P. Gunnemann

How we—any of us—understand justice in health care rests in large measure on how we understand health care. What sort of good is health care? In the twenty-first-century United States, health care is framed in multiple and sometimes overlapping ways: Health care is a social good, public work, and civic practice, a commodity, a private benefit, a professional service, or, in more explicitly moral terms, a human right, as well as an individual or social responsibility.[1] Here I focus on health care as a particular type of social good, that is, as a community good. The implications of this understanding for health care justice are substantial. To the extent that we understand health care as a community good, then justice in health care must engage the community dimensions of health care.

To say that health care is a social good is to say that it is fundamentally relational. In health care ethics, and particularly in the discourse of justice in health care, to say that health care is a social good typically means that health care is a national or societal good. The relational scope of health is assumed to be the society, and justice is often framed around the question of whether society (or the nation) has responsibility in the provision of health care to its members.

In this book I bring a different lens to the notion of health care as a social good, one that begins with the recognition that health care is social at many levels of collectivity: interpersonal, family, community, state, nation-society, international, and transnational-global. Communities, I argue, are the primary, but not exclusive, contexts for the social relations and institutions most central to U.S. health care. Most social interactions critical to health care occur within various communities, including local neighborhoods, towns, and cities; religious communities; cultural, racial, and ethnic communities; and school, work, and professional communities. As becomes clear, these diverse types of communities tend to play different and multivalent roles in health care.

On Community

The term "community" has many meanings, and its definitions, scopes, characteristics, and taxonomies have been the subject of much attention and contestation across academic disciplines, in the professional realms of public health and health promotion, as well as in community organizing. Often the notion of community is portrayed as slippery or messy. Calling communities "restless and unruly," Michael Gross notes how serious and critical attention to communities "shatters the normative monism imposed by liberalism."[2] He observes, "Herein lies the sloppiness that communities bring to medicine. The normative directions are now less clear-cut, less universal, and less focused on the individual as patient. Conflicting norms and players compete with one another, bringing a measure of chaos to medical decisionmaking."[3] Perhaps this perceived unruliness of communities has contributed to the weak presence of communities in much of contemporary bioethical analysis, an absence noted by feminist bioethicists at least two decades ago.[4] This restlessness is not, I suggest, an obstacle to clear moral reflection or reasoning but, rather, a welcome, even necessary condition for the creation of a more inclusive and respectful concept of justice for health care.

I begin with the familiar understanding that communities are a type of social group and add that such a group "may be more or less of a community."[5] In *The Moral Commonwealth: Social Theory and the Promise of Community*, Philip Selznick elaborates on the features of community: "A group is a community to the extent that it encompasses a broad range of activities and interests, and to the extent that participation implicates whole persons rather than segmental interests or activities." As such, "the emergence of a community depends on the opportunity for, and the impulse toward, comprehensive interaction, commitment, and responsibility."[6] In this meaning of community, which I adopt here, communities are relatively wide and deep social groups: The more extensive the shared activities and the more wholly that group members participate in, identify with, and take responsibility for the group, the stronger is its community nature. Groups that live and work together—for example, some religious and military groups—are likely to be relatively strong communities compared to groups that form solely, say, to watch birds or play soccer. A collection of persons waiting for a bus on a given day would rarely constitute a community or even a group in some definitions.[7] As the theologian John Cobb observes, "The more responsibility the members take for one another, whether expressed directly or indirectly, the more of a community it will be. The more strongly people identify themselves by their membership, the more the community functions as a community. And the more members perceive themselves as full participants in the life and decision-making of the group, the more truly it is a community."[8] Thus communities exist on a spectrum of weak to strong depending on the identification, participation, and mutual responsibility of their members. Since no bright line exists between social groups and communities, I sometimes use these terms interchangeably.

Such academic understandings of community sometimes align with popular meanings. A qualitative public health study of potential community collaboration related to HIV vaccine trials found that diverse participants, including African Americans in North Carolina, injection drug users in Pennsylvania, and HIV vaccine researchers across the United States, share a largely common understanding of community distilled as "*a group of people with diverse characteristics who are linked by social ties, share common perspectives, and engage in joint action in geographical locations or settings.*"[9] Each of five core elements of this definition of community—locus, sharing, joint action, social ties, and diversity—were differentially important for the various groups of research participants, signaling that the groups' experience community differently. That said, their understandings of community overlap significantly and echo those in the scholarly literature.

Communities are sometimes represented as different than society writ large. The *Oxford English Dictionary* defines community as a "group of people who share the same interests, pursuits, or occupation, esp. when distinct from those of the society in which they live."[10] Yet if communities are both distinct from society and live in society, who is society? I address this relationship between society and communities in detail later. For now, I embrace a social ontology in which society is composed of many diverse groups and communities that interact with one another and with larger and smaller collectivities, all with varying degrees of influence and power. In this perspective, there is no generic or unified society apart from distinct communities, only a society made up of many particular communities in complex interaction.

Very different social collectivities with distinct membership criteria can rightfully be called communities. Communities may share place, history, experience, goals, projects, religion, culture, ethnicity, race, social class, gender, sexuality, ability, age, illness, occupation, and more. The elderly, the middle class, the medical profession, evangelical Christians, local geopolitical communities, African Americans, the LGBTQ (lesbian, gay, bisexual, trans, and queer) community, the disability community, the breast cancer survivor community—these are just a few of the communities that shape the health and health care of both community members and noncommunity members. Importantly, most persons are members of multiple communities—often "competing value-creating communities"—that create and hold plural values and understandings about health care and related social goods.[11]

Notably, communities, which by definition share something in common, are not uniform in belief or membership.[12] Not all community members identify with or participate in that particular commonality to the same degree, and member identification and participation can shift over time. Communities are rarely discrete, tidy units; rather, they typically have porous and shifting boundaries. Communities are often parts of larger regional, societal, national, and global social collectivities and simultaneously are composed of smaller diverse communities. For example, the Asian American community in Los Angeles is nested within larger state and regional Asian American communities and at the same time includes Chinese, Thai, Japanese, and Vietnamese communities across the spectra of social class and immigration status. Each of these communities, too, is nested within larger state and regional culture-specific communities.

Additionally, communities are inextricably tied to family relations and to societal and national contexts. In health and health care this has increasingly become the case as health care providers have merged and consolidated, moving from local to national and transnational institutions, and as families and communities have taken on more care of sick family members as the length of hospital stays has declined.

Perhaps most important, communities have varying degrees of power, voice, and stability. Physicians have considerably more power in defining and treating health and disease than, say, nurse practitioners or Christian Scientists.

Local geographic communities provide more solid ground, literally and figuratively, for the delivery of health care services than does, say, an age-based community. Power operates within each community as well, making for varying degrees of inclusion or marginalization of community members. Communities are not essentially traditional or progressive, or even repressive or liberative, though they can function in all these and other ways. Communities are diverse, interdependent, dynamic, "messy," and fundamentally salient to just health care.

Communities are related critically to health and health care in (at least) four ways: (1) Communities are *meaning making*: it is in communities that we learn, create, re-create, and negotiate particular understandings of health, illness, and health care. (2) Communities literally shape the *health* of their members. (3) *Health care* often takes place in community contexts. (4) And communities themselves *benefit* from (or are harmed by) health care activities and institutions. The rest of this chapter elaborates on these four community dimensions of health care, dimensions that justice in health care must account for.

Communities as Sites of Meaning Making

The meanings we give to health, illness, healing, health care, and death are not created de novo. We are born into and join communities with diverse and normative traditions, cultures, practices, and values that shape our individual understandings of the nature of health, disease, and healing. And we participate in the ongoing social processes of reshaping those community meanings and norms. The following illustrations of communities are not comprehensive; rather, they reveal the wide-ranging and diverse health-related meaning-making communities present in the United States today. This pluralism of meanings can be difficult to perceive given the power, or more precisely, the supremacy, of the biomedical community as the authoritative definer of health and disease. Rooted in a scientific European heritage and developed in the nineteenth-century United States by the professional community of "regular" or allopathic physicians, biomedicine emerged in the context of and in opposition to the panoply of "irregular" healing practitioners of the time.[13] Generally speaking, biomedical culture emphasizes disease and treatment of the individual physical body; it understands healing as curing, health as the absence of disease, and prevention as secondary to treatment. The core tenets of biomedicine are so deeply embedded in everyday thinking as to be assumed by many persons. These tenets include the belief that disease is a deviation from some biological or functional norm; that disease has a singular and specific etiology or cause (usually a pathogen); that diseases are ahistorical realities—that is, they are unchanging across time and space; and, finally, that medicine, like science, is objective in the sense of being impartial.[14] Naming these foundational biomedical principles reveals biomedicine to be hardly neutral but rather one type of cultural medicine, one specific healing system, that emerges from a particular history and social location and that reaffirms a particular set of social and cultural values. As Elizabeth Fee and Nancy Krieger argue, "Ultimately, the biomedical model embodies an approach to analyzing disease that is fundamentally individualistic and sanctions only the physicians' or scientists' point of view. Profoundly ahistorical, it contains within itself a dichotomy between the biological individual and the social community, and then it ignores the latter."[15]

The contemporary biomedical community transcends the U.S. context and yet is shaped by it.[16] Though biomedical practice within a nation tends to exhibit similar general characteristics, substantial variation in physician practice exists by geographic area, reflecting the development of not only regional but also rather localized norms of practice. Atul Gawande's widely read 2009 *New Yorker* article compares health care outcomes and costs in two Texas towns, bringing the reality of differences in community-level medical practice to national attention as well as to health care reform discussions.[17] Earlier 1980s work by Dartmouth Medical School's Center for the Evaluative Clinical Sciences revealed strikingly different patterns of health care utilization by locality across the nation, leading the study's authors to declare in 1996 that, "in health care markets, geography is destiny: the care one receives depends in large part on the supply of resources available in the place where one lives— and on the practice patterns of local physicians."[18]

Elliot Mishler rightly observes that in the United States biomedicine "is treated as *the* representation or picture of reality rather than understood as *a* representation."[19] The medical profession is an "epistemic community" and as a profession has been granted "the official power to define and therefore create the shape of problematic segments of social behavior: the judge determines what is legal and who is guilty, the priest what is holy and who is profane, the physician what is normal and who is sick."[20] By collective professional decision, biomedicine defines particular conditions in, and occasionally out of, disease status. Over the course of the last century, pregnancy and childbirth, menopause, dying, and, more recently, gender identity, shortness of stature, and sexual desire have been medicalized and brought under the authority and definition of the biomedical community.[21] Collins O. Airhihenbuwa names such biomedical control "allopathic hegemony" and asserts that biomedicine's understandings, while dominant, are not absolute, nor is biomedicine's authority unchallenged.[22]

Beyond the definitions of health and disease and the health care practices established by the biomedical community, meaning making regarding health and health care also takes place in many and diverse cultural and religious communities.[23] Indigenous Native American communities have created forms of traditional medicine that understand persons and their health as essentially relational, spiritual, and communal in contrast to the more individualistic, biological orientation of biomedicine.[24] In these indigenous worldviews, generally speaking, health is not the absence of disease but, rather, a matter of harmony and balance within oneself and with family, communities, and the cosmos. Some indigenous Hawaiian communities understand that persons and the Earth are interdependent and that nature itself can be a healing agent.[25] Mid-nineteenth-century Chinese immigrants to the United States brought healing systems born of Buddhist, Confucian, and Taoist beliefs and traditions, including healing practices involving acupuncture, medicinal herbs, *qigong*, and more.[26]

Certain Black communities in the United States embody systems of healing beliefs and practices that reflect an integrated understanding of health as having physical, mental, and spiritual components. In tandem, disease is understood as having individual biological origins as well as social causes rooted in racism and a legacy of slavery.[27] Building on the notion of health as a cultural production, Emilie M. Townes challenges the African American community "to recognize and engage what health as a cultural production means in Black cultures, which are dynamic processes constantly interpreting and reinterpreting values, beliefs, norms, and practices—consciously and unconsciously."[28] In documenting these cultural productions for over a decade, the Boston Healing Landscape Project mapped and thus made visible the diverse cultural and religious healing traditions of communities of the African Diaspora (as well as other communities) in the Boston area.[29]

Healing is centrally important to the theology and practice of the First Church of Christ, Scientist, commonly known as the Christian Science Church. In contrast to adherents of biomedicine, Christian Scientists understand illness, not as an objective pathogen-based reality, but rather as a condition manifest and strengthened by one's belief in the condition. Healing authority is found in Mary Baker Eddy's *Science and Health, with Key to the Scriptures*, and healing itself is achieved through prayer and scripture reading rather than through either a physician's clinical judgment or pharmacology.[30]

Important health-related meaning making also takes place in and among less discretely identifiable social groups—for example, those marked by gender and ability. Motivated by medicine's historical neglect of women's understandings of health and health care needs, women, largely through the women's health movement, have succeeded somewhat in redefining common ideas about health and health care. For example, women's health activists (largely cis-gendered) have worked to demedicalize childbirth and menopause; to promote the idea that "domestic" violence, like street violence, is a public health problem; and to convince health officials and lawmakers that access to contraception is critical to health. Some health activists work to redefine entrenched social norms about gender and thus to reduce the neglect of transgender and gender-variant persons in research and clinical services. They challenge the conventional gender binary—the idea that there are two essential genders, man and woman—and promote an understanding of gender that embraces persons whose gender identity shifts between these conventional genders as well as persons who do not identify with any gender. The gender binary limits our ability to accurately diagnose and treat persons who do not fit that gender frame and promotes pathologizing them. Changes in biomedical practice are evident in the reduction of gender-conforming surgeries done on newborns and in the development of hormone therapies and later-in-life gender-affirming surgeries.

Through the disability rights movement, disabled persons have developed, embraced, and spread new ways of thinking about ability and disability. In particular, they have advanced the realization that disability is created through a lack of access and accommodation and thus is a social rather than simply an individual and biomedical concern. At the same time, they have challenged the notion of dependency as atypical and problematic and argued that most persons live interdependently with others, experiencing greater and lesser degrees of dependency throughout one's lifetime.

Many health beliefs and practices result from the blending of different healing cultures and systems, including biomedicine. Jehovah's Witnesses are well known to hospital personnel, not because they rebuff biomedicine in general, but because they strongly reject a particular biomedical therapy, the blood transfusion. Hmong understandings of health and healing have been popularized in Ann Fadiman's *The Spirit Catches You and You Fall Down*, the tragic story of a Hmong family's efforts to hold onto their cultural understandings and practices within the U.S. biomedical context.[31] In the course of describing her life as a Navajo woman, mother, and surgeon, Lori Arviso Alvord, in her autobiographical narrative, *The Scalpel and the Silver Bear*, explains the health-related meanings of the Diné people—and their lessons for contemporary biomedicine, thus reversing the typical epistemic dynamic between biomedicine and other forms of cultural healing.[32]

Not only does collective meaning making define health and healing, but the social process of meaning making itself can be a form of community building and community healing. For example, the restoration or re-creation of indigenous cultural identity through food practices, storytelling, and healing rituals resists ongoing cultural assimilation (neocolonialism) and can strengthen one's sense of self and healthy relations within the community.[33]

The processes of community meaning making are vibrant and ongoing, and conceptions of health and health care are continually being reshaped by influences both internal and external to particular communities. It is notable that, although meanings are often created in particular communities, they also affect others outside those communities. Multiple meanings coexist and interact as communities share members and otherwise associate with one another, especially in a society as heterogeneous as that of the United States.

Community Factors in Health

Health is in large measure the result of physical and social macro environments at the local community level. The local physical environment—including, for example, air, water, and soil quality; climate; noise levels; toxins; and housing and transportation patterns—is commonly understood to affect human health. This physical environment, however, is deeply intertwined with the social environment, that is, with social relations, the integration of which has come to be known in the health arena as "place." As Steven Cummins and colleagues put it, "Place is relevant for health variation because it *constitutes* as well as *contains* social relations and physical resources."[34]

Contagion is a classic example of the interpersonal relational nature of health or, more precisely, of sickness. We literally share disease and health with one another. Infectious diseases such as influenza and tuberculosis spread primarily among persons living or working in close proximity to one another, as in homes, schools, day care centers, hospitals, stores, shelters, and worksites. Other infectious diseases are transmitted by more direct social relations, for example, by sexual contact. Thus contagion is largely a feature of in-person communities, that is, communities bound at least in part by place. That said, the global reaches—actual and potential—of Ebola, human immunodeficiency virus (HIV), and tuberculosis show just how fluid and connected communities are.

Over the last three decades, social epidemiology and related work have made evident the many social determinants that influence health and disease in populations from the neighborhood to the global level.[35] Studies of neighborhood and community factors, observes David Williams, constitute the current era of epidemiological research.[36] Income and wealth, education, job opportunities and working conditions, race and other social group relations, food (in)security, and migration are among the fundamental and complexly intersecting conditions that lead to significant health consequences.

Interpersonal social relations within and among communities shape health. Family, friendship, marriage, and religious community membership and other group affiliations are generally beneficial to health, though the benefits vary by gender and race. The cultural production of health is illustrated by the Latin@ health paradox, where Latin@s with relatively low social class status and strong, culturally promoted health behaviors have lower mortality rates compared to non-Latin@ whites.[37] In general, less socially integrated persons have a significantly greater risk of mortality and perhaps of morbidity. Violence has a negative health effect not only on its immediate victims and witnesses but also on the social cohesion of communities as a whole. Discrimination, marginalization, and other forms of oppression—whether based on race, gender, immigration status, or other factors—contribute to social stress and negatively affect health. In contrast, structural pluralism, defined as "the degree to which organizations and population segments of a community have the capacity to participate in political exchange," has been shown to be predictive of lower mortality.[38] Communal stability, support, and social solidarity positively affect health through the promotion of social cohesion and community engagement and participation.[39]

As Linda M. Burton and her colleagues observe, place "is more than a spatial backdrop for social interaction or a proxy for neighborhood variables. Place is a socio-ecological force" that "reflect[s] and reinforce[s] social advantages and disadvantages" and serves as a conduit for "segregation, marginalization, collective action" and other social processes such as displacement and detachment.[40] In short, those who constitute a community demographically—by age, gender, ethnicity, and social class—and how these community members relate to one another significantly condition their health.

Community-Based Health Care

As noted earlier, health care is essentially a social relationship. Care, as described by bioethicist Daniel Callahan, is "a positive emotional and supportive response to the condition and situation of another person, a response whose purpose is to affirm our commitment to their well-being, our willingness to identify with them in their pain and suffering, and our desire to do what we can do to relieve their situation."[41] As a positive commitment to help at least some ill or injured persons in need of healing, health care has interpersonal and institutional dimensions, both of which exist most often and most intensely in one's local community setting. A person's suffering and need for care affect most significantly the members of one's most immediate and local relations. These include people in the ill person's family, workplaces, and community-based health care institutions.

Sheer proximity may evoke caring or a commitment to some level of attention and responsibility. In 2013, 82 percent of U.S. adults surveyed said they care about the health of their neighbors, suggesting high-level attention to the suffering and needs of those with whom we feel some common bond of place or interaction.[42]

Local communities in the United States have long played multiple roles in health care.[43] Beginning in the mid-1800s, community hospitals were established to care for local residents as well as to train physicians and nurses. Some religious and ethnic immigrant communities set up hospitals to care for their community members who were, at times, excluded from local community hospitals as patients or as physicians. In the early 1900s, mutual aid associations created by culturally specific immigrant groups, "fraternal" orders, and employee associations contracted with physicians to provide services to their members. This collective pooling of financial risk enabled members to receive otherwise unaffordable care. Community rating served as the prototype for health insurance, which would blossom in the 1930s and 1940s. Similarly, prepaid group health plans, the precursors of health maintenance organizations, were established to enable a defined group to receive care.

By the late 1960s and early 1970s, hundreds of local communities had established neighborhood health centers in response to the health care needs of low-income persons as well as the desire for community governance. "Free clinics" run by local practitioners and medical students including the People's Free Medical Clinics of the Black Panther Party were initiated in this period, as were feminist health centers.[44] Today, community-based safety net providers, including community health centers and local nonprofit hospitals, care for many uninsured persons, while employers and state exchanges are the primary providers of health plans, and thus access to health care, to insured persons. Substantial medical training and research take place in academic medical centers, revealing some of the benefits these communities offer to medical and other health care professionals.

Among religious communities in the United States, health care is most prominent in the work of the U.S. Catholic Church, as evidenced by its more than two thousand hospitals and long-term care and other health facilities, its active engagement in health policy, and its substantial meaning-making influence. Church teachings promote particular understandings—of the person, of the community, and of medical and sexual ethics—that shape how Catholics think about what constitutes a healthy and good life. Moreover, these meanings and values determine the practices of Catholic health care facilities, which serve both Catholics and non-Catholics. Best known are those values prohibiting medical services related to sexual and reproductive health—abortion, sterilization, contraception, and condom promotion—and those promoting spiritual well-being and access to care for the medically underserved.

Owing to the strong influence of the biomedical community, health *care* is often understood as the interaction between trained professionals and patients in the context of a clinic, physician's office, or hospital. The dyadic image of physician-patient care obscures the extensive institutional and interpersonal network necessary for a caring healing encounter to occur. A simple primary-care visit is likely to require that a patient engage face to face with a receptionist, a billing clerk, a physician or nurse practitioner, a nurse or a medical assistant, and perhaps laboratory and pharmacy personnel—in addition to multiple other "invisible" employees of the institution that make this care possible.

This patient-practitioner relationship is set within a complex set of organizational contexts that either enhance or constrain care. "The organizational and administrative (not to mention cultural) contexts in which doctors and patients interact crucially affect the ability of each to act toward the other in a caring fashion," argues one group of commentators. Specifically, they find that the "relational distance" between health care practitioners and patients is importantly influenced by the organizational context.[45]

Additionally, professional care givers typically practice within a local professional community with particular standards of practice and are members of local and state professional associations. They are strongly influenced by the mores, views, and practices of their colleagues—from the services they provide, to the equipment and techniques they use, to the medicines they prescribe. Physicians and others are also subject to legal standards regarding practitioner authority, permitted practices, and professional relations.

Neglected in this focus on the professional, formal system of care is the extensive network of care typically given by family, friends, neighbors, and other community members. Parents (often mothers), adult children (often daughters and daughters-in-law), neighbors, friends, and other loved ones provide substantial care in the home and, increasingly, also in hospitals and nursing homes, as the attention of institutional health care providers is divided by multiple demands. Needy persons, especially those with chronic illnesses, are often cared for by communities with which they feel a sense of belonging. Critically, this often-obscured care work relies almost exclusively on the social networks of particular communities—familial, cultural, religious, or disease experience oriented.

Persons experiencing a particular health condition or disease often join with others with like experiences and needs to advocate for themselves. The recent growth in number, size, and activism of illness communities—face-to-face and virtual—reflects the experience that having a particular condition or need can bond otherwise strangers in their search for appropriate attention and care.[46] For example, the heterogeneous communities most affected by HIV have long organized to create effective prevention strategies, care for persons with HIV and AIDS, and demand improved and more accessible treatment options.[47]

In all these and other important ways, health care—the care of health—takes place in a wide range of communities both inside and outside of conventional health care facilities.

Community Benefits of Health Care

While individual community members receive benefits from health care, communities as a whole also benefit. Health care institutions support other community institutions by helping to keep individual community members healthy and capable of contributing to those institutions as workers, students, and political participants. As noted above, for some indigenous communities, respectful healing practices can contribute to cultural healing and even cultural survival.[48]

Nonprofit and public hospitals, like similarly owned universities and colleges (known as "eds and meds"), have the potential to be anchor institutions in local communities, according to David Zuckerman, author of "Hospitals Building Healthier Communities: Embracing the Anchor Mission." These hospitals with "their expanding economic impact and connection to their locations [are] strategically position[ed] . . . to produce targeted community benefits if they leverage their resources effectively."[49] A 2015 *New York Times* article,

"Hospitals Provide a Pulse in Struggling Rural Towns," by Dionne Searcey, features Beatrice, Nebraska, a town with a population of approximately twelve thousand some forty miles from the state capital. Its new nonprofit Beatrice Community Hospital and Health Center is "an essential economic engine" of that town, sustained in part by enhanced Medicare reimbursement due to its status as a critical access hospital. Such thriving hospitals, "beyond providing an array of jobs from the bottom to the top of the economic ladder, also stimulate local spending and help attract new businesses that offer a stable of insured patients."[50]

Such health care institutions are integral to the institutional fabric of local community life and have the potential to strengthen community infrastructure not only economically but also through providing educational training and leadership opportunities. Community participation in local health care institutions in advisory or governance capacities, for example, may promote broader democratic political involvement. As such, health care institutions have the potential to contribute to social solidarity and cohesion as well as to social stress and disorganization.

Historically, mutual aid societies sponsored health care services for their members—and as a result strengthened their communities as a whole. Since the late 1960s, the promotion of community participation in community health centers has been a modestly effective means of bringing new voices and values to community health governance. More recently, the Patient Protection and Affordable Care Act of 2010 (ACA) mandates that nonprofit hospitals report their community benefits activities as well as engage with public health officials and community members to complete a triennial community health needs assessment and a corresponding plan for community health improvement.

Health care is in large measure a community good, dependent on the social relations located in multiple and diverse subnational communities. It is primarily in these communities that the meanings of health and health care are created, negotiated, and shared; that people are made healthy and sick; that care is given and received; and that the benefits of health care are accrued. This description of the community dimensions of health care also suggests that different types of communities tend to make characteristic but not exclusive kinds of contributions to health and health care. Cultural and religious communities, for example, are particularly important as sites of health-related meaning making—that is, as sources of understandings about health and health care—and certain of these communities also provide important health care institutions and social support. Local communities or places encompass the physical environments and social relations of the multiple constitutive communities that are determinative of health. Health care is a positive response to persons in need of healing and is typically offered by local community providers in these local places. Communities of all types benefit from health care, as do individuals, families, and the larger society.

Recall what is at stake in this recognition of health care as a community good: how we think about a good shapes how we think about justice in relation to that good. To the extent that health care is a community good, our understanding of justice in health care must embrace these community dimensions.

Chapter 2

Communities Obscured

Liberal Theories of Health Care Justice

Generally speaking, liberal theories of justice in health care guide normative relations between individuals and society, as they center on individuals and society as the justice-relevant moral entities. Despite the multiple and important roles that diverse communities play in health and health care, these theories grant little attention, and even less positive moral significance, to communities. Yet justice in health care must account for communities—as meaning makers, as contributors to health, as providers of health care (interpersonal and institutional), and as recipients of health care's benefits—and in chapter 4 I argue constructively for a concept of community justice that attempts to do that. In this chapter, I examine the communities and their moral roles found within six egalitarian and capability theories of health care justice, theories chosen because they are critical, well-developed frameworks, prominent in bioethical discourse about justice in health care, and have the potential to influence relevant actors directly through public bioethics venues or indirectly through the education of policy makers, bioethicists, and health care practitioners.[1]

This inquiry finds that not only do communities receive minimal consideration in these theories overall but the communities that are recognized tend to be clustered either as religious or cultural communities or as groups bound by race, gender, or social class. As to their moral roles, religious and cultural communities are typically represented as threats or obstacles to justice in health care, whereas communities defined by race, gender, or class tend to be portrayed as disadvantaged, vulnerable, and largely morally irrelevant to just health care. Advantaged, dominant, or "majority" communities are remarkably unmarked—that is to say, seldom explicitly acknowledged—and the same holds for their moral roles as communities. This analysis establishes the clear need for a new and different conversation about communities and health care justice. Making visible the precise ways that these theories morally marginal-ize communities is instructive for avoiding such marginalization in crafting an alternate multilayered, relational, and inclusive theory of justice in health care.

Communities as Threats and Obstacles

Egalitarian theories of justice, represented here by Norman Daniels's theory of just health, Leonard Fleck's just caring framework, and Shlomi Segall's luck egalitarianism,[2] tend to characterize communities and their members as chal-lenges to the rational, democratic deliberation they understand as necessary for just health care. As egalitarian theories, they generally coincide in their fundamental assumptions about the nature of individuals and of society and in their attention to just decision making in a deliberative democracy. As such, the scope of justice is typically the aggregate members of a nation-state.

Daniels offers a theory of just population health that "tell[s] us what we owe each other in the protection and promotion of health."[3] Health, he asserts, is morally important because it influences life's opportunities. Health inequalities contribute to opportunity inequalities and are unjust if they result from "an unjust distribution of the socially controllable factors."[4] Even persons who agree with this substantive understanding of health justice rea-sonably disagree about how to allocate limited health resources fairly. Thus Daniels argues that just health requires a fair deliberative process for resource allocation, a process that abides by four criteria to assure "accountability for reasonableness."[5]

Although attending primarily to the U.S. population as a whole, Daniels references principally two sorts of communities: vulnerable population sub-groups, and religious and cultural communities. He recognizes population subgroups defined by social class, gender, race, and ethnicity that experience health and social inequalities rooted in social discrimination.[6] Blacks and women, he notes, experience discrimination that constrains their access to myriad social conditions that promote health, for example, adequate income, education, and housing. Such discrimination reduces health status, access to health care, and, ultimately, life opportunities.[7] Acknowledging this dispropor-tionate vulnerability and exclusion, Daniels allows that the unjust inequality of groups "may justify giving some extra priority to the worst off," though finally it remains individuals, not communities or groups, that are granted moral pri-ority or salience.[8]

In contrast, Daniels situates religious and cultural communities as potential or actual sources of injustice in two ways. First, he notes that the social inequalities experienced by vulnerable subgroups defined by gender, race, and class are created in part by religious and cultural communities: Social inequalities are "significantly affected by bias associated with cultural and religious practices."[9] More specifically, opportunity is thwarted by "gender-based attitudes, with their deep cultural and religious roots."[10]

The second way religious and cultural communities are deemed problematic for justice is found in Daniels's fourfold conditions for accountability for reasonableness. Established to ensure a fair process of resource allocation, these conditions stipulate that allocation decisions and their rationales or reasons must be made publicly accessible, that is, they must be made in public; they must be relevant; they must be revisable; and they must be regulated. "Reasons," says Daniels, "must reflect the fact that all parties to a decision are viewed as seeking terms of fair cooperation that all can accept as reasonable. Where their well-being and fundamental liberties or other matters of fundamental value are involved and at risk, people should not be expected to accept binding terms of cooperation that rest on types of reasons they find unacceptable. For example, reasons that rest on matters of religious faith will not meet this condition."[11] Daniels allows that different persons will prioritize evidence and principles differently and that the fair decision-making processes of different groups will have different outcomes. Nonetheless, relevant rationales are "ones that all stakeholders should accept as relevant and appropriate," making religious rationales irrelevant and thus inadmissible in public deliberation related to health care decision making.[12]

Concurrently, Daniels affirms that "the giving of reasons must itself respect the moral diversity of those affected by the decisions," setting up a strong tension between these two claims about the nature of a fair decision-making process.[13] On the one hand, reasons and rationales must be recognized as relevant and appropriate by all stakeholders understood as "('fair-minded') people who are disposed to finding mutually justifiable terms of cooperation."[14] On the other hand, the decision-making process must respect the moral diversity of participants. Daniels reveals his prioritization of universal relevance over respect for diversity in his designation of universal relevance as a necessary condition for decision making while granting no such standing for respect for moral diversity.

Several critical questions arise here. Are any worldviews—philosophical, theological, or other—relevant and accessible to all nonadherents? Is it "reasonable" to introduce to democratic deliberation only rationales that some deem relevant and appropriate? Might not fair-minded people *want* to engage, understand, discuss, and deliberate a wider range of perspectives, including some that they, at least initially, might not believe to be relevant or reasonable? Might not a fair decision-making process be enhanced by more and diverse perspectives, especially in a population characterized by social and health inequities and marginalized subgroups?

Furthermore, in this theory community-based meanings and values are set aside in (at least) two additional ways. The first is embedded in the claim that the special moral importance of health is its effects on opportunity. Daniels explains, "I am not giving an anthropological explanation that says that people believe health protects opportunity and they value opportunity. If asked, people may say that they think health care is important for many reasons, including the fact that it saves lives or reduces suffering. My explanation reflects people's *real* interests and coheres well with the justification for thinking that meeting health needs is morally important, namely, that we have an obligation to protect opportunity and that protecting health protects opportunity."[15] Thus Daniels recognizes that people may hold different ideas about the moral importance of health and still asserts a singular understanding, thus masking not only the diverse meanings about health that people may actually hold but also the cultural, religious, and other communities within which these meanings are formed and maintained.

Another trumping of community understandings and values by the principle of fair equality of opportunity is evident in Daniels's critique of Michael Walzer's account of complex equality. Whereas Walzer allows that societies may justly prioritize values—for example, spiritual salvation—over physical health and opportunity,[16] Daniels argues that it is unjust to fail to protect health and thus opportunity when a society could reasonably do so.[17] Again, the principle of equality of opportunity is asserted to outweigh the multiple and diverse priorities, meanings, and values embraced by multiple and diverse groups.

On the whole, in this account communities are not recognized as morally relevant to just health care except as vulnerable population subgroup members who may warrant priority in just allocation decisions and as certain religious community members who may risk impeding fair decision-making processes with irrelevant rationales. This marginalization of communities is especially notable in light of Daniels's attention to global justice and in particular to his exploration of "a middle ground" between nation-states' views and cosmopolitan individualism.[18] He envisions a relational, "multilayered construction" of international justice in which the principles of justice rest with "middle ground" intermediary institutions between nation-states and the global citizenry, that is, with "recently formed and evolving international agencies, institutions, and rule-making bodies."[19] In this global scope, Daniels recognizes intermediate social collectivities as morally vital. But in the national scope, his account of just health does not offer a multilayered construction of justice inclusive of morally necessary intermediate collectivities—that is, inclusive of the communities and groups that reside between individuals and nation-states.[20]

Fleck's egalitarian theory of health care justice parallels Daniels's account in significant ways, and to the extent that communities are evident, it, too, recognizes primarily religious, cultural, and marginalized communities, though with different emphases. In Fleck's framework, just health care must respond to the problem of fair rationing of limited health care resources. In a liberal society whose members hold many diverse ideas of justice, no one idea can legitimately serve as *the* distributive principle for resource allocation, so Fleck adopts a procedural approach to justice he calls "just caring." Just caring is a process of rational and principled democratic deliberation with the goal "to create rules or policies or practices . . . that all will have to live with and that are fair and reasonable."[21] "Citizen deliberators" are assumed to be free and equal persons who want to sustain a liberal, pluralistic society "in which we are all cooperative, mutually respectful members."[22] For democratic deliberation, individual differences in, for example, social class and education, are deemed irrelevant. This deliberative process requires that its participants give public reasons for their perspectives—that is, reasons tied to the public or common interest understood as universally valued. Notably, these public reasons must be detached from religious worldviews or specific metaphysical perspectives.

Fleck contends that we must address health care rationing at multiple levels of the social context: at the societal level, at the level of health care institutions and organizations, and at the patient care level.[23] Notably, communities are not among those social contexts. In Fleck's view, individuals in their roles as society members are the moral entities most important to democratic deliberation. Society members who are also members of religious communities—Jehovah's Witnesses, Christian Scientists, Roman Catholics, and Muslims—are sources of concern: concern that their deeply held beliefs might interrupt fair processes of public deliberation.

Fleck posits eight fundamental and necessary "constitutional principles" of health care justice and rational democratic deliberation not unlike Daniels's criteria of accountability for reasonableness. In important ways, two of the eight principles—liberal neutrality, and respect for persons—involve communities. Liberal neutrality requires that public reasons be given to justify health care rationing protocols. These reasons cannot appeal to "moral or metaphysical" truths, for these truths are understood to be inherently partisan and biased.[24] Public reason's vital role, according to Fleck, is to provide a framework strong enough to hold within it—and to hold together—society with its often profoundly conflicting beliefs and commitments. Fleck maintains that deliberators who hold comprehensive philosophic or religious worldviews must find, within such views, values that are "neutral or agnostic with respect to the truth claims of those doctrines," and these deliberators must bring only those values that "transcend all comprehensive doctrines" to the table of democratic deliberation.[25]

Fleck recognizes that communities are vital meaning makers, shaping members' health care values and needs in particular ways. For Fleck these particularities create "the liberalism problem": the challenge of a neutral liberal society committed to universal public reason to justly treat "particular" persons. In *Just Caring*, Fleck repeatedly uses religious communities to illustrate hypothetical violations of liberal neutrality and public reason: A psychiatrist tells a patient questioning his gender identity that their therapeutic session will not be covered by insurance because "the substance of this conversation is deeply offensive to more conservative religious sects in our society"; public funding for biomedical care is suspended "to avoid giving offense to Christian Scientists" who ascribe to a spiritual healing system; and a national health plan refuses to pay for pregnancy-related counseling that includes speaking of abortion owing to opposition from the Catholic Church.[26] In these examples, religious views are not only represented as challenges to public reason, they lead to the denial of needed care. In the absence of positive or affirming comments involving religion, this positioning of religious communities as sources of potential violations of liberal neutrality and democracy reasonably suggests a skepticism, if not outright distrust, of these communities and their community members.

This wariness is also reflected in a second principle of democratic deliberation: respect for persons. This principle requires "respect for cultural and religious differences among patients related to health care needs"—within limits: "Our general social rule (as a liberal, pluralistic society) ought to be seeking to accommodate special health care needs related to the cultural or religious commitments of patients *so long as the accommodation of those needs does not threaten the just claims of other patients to have their health needs met."*[27] Two points are in order here. First, note that culturally and religiously related health care needs are understood and labeled as *special* needs, thus distinguished from general or ordinary health care needs, as if all health care needs are not at least in part socially or culturally particular. As noted in chapter 1, biomedicine, too, is a particular medical culture that defines health needs in a particular way. Second, accommodating religious and cultural needs only when they do not "threaten" nonreligious and cultural needs relegates these special needs to a secondary tier of moral importance. Given the overall and abiding gap in health care resources relative to needs, all needs in effect "threaten" each other. It is unclear how downgrading religiously and culturally related needs relative to other needs honors the principle of respect for persons.

Fleck here again uses members of religious communities to exemplify a violation of public reason, in this case, a violation of respect for persons. He argues that Jehovah's Witnesses can refuse blood transfusions and can justly ask for modified surgical interventions. But they are not entitled to a costly blood-clotting drug at public expense because that care might the limit resources for others' more deserved needs, in other words, for those with fewer "special" needs. This does not disrespect Jehovah's Witnesses, says Fleck; rather, it is a consequence of our liberal commitments to respect diverse religious views by insisting that we will not provide public subsidies for the support of an individual's religious beliefs, especially when they are provided at the expense of other just health care claims.[28] To provide such public support would be both "unjust and illiberal," claims Fleck.[29] Instead, religious communities themselves are responsible for caring for their members' medical needs if they are related to religious and cultural commitments.

Standing in seeming contrast to the above marginalizing representations of communities, Fleck relates his experiences directing health-related public deliberative forums in the 1980s and 1990s. One such forum specifically engaged communities of color on issues of genetics and public policy.[30] In a seeming challenge to the principle of liberal neutrality, Fleck intentionally recruited a wide range of likely quite partial deliberation partners—"from Right to Life, various religious groups, and various disability groups"—into these public deliberative forums.[31] Those deliberative experiences led him to assert a "critical requirement" of deliberation: "These deliberative groups [must] be broadly representative of all those who will be affected by the priority-setting process, especially those social groups that are least well off and most often excluded from effective participation in democratic politics. This is a very demanding requirement but it is a matter of absolute necessity."[32]

Were these group representatives invited to participate but then asked to leave their deeply rooted moral beliefs and motivations, whether religious, cultural, or philosophical, at the door? Were they allowed to present and engage only with values that were "neutral or agnostic with respect to the truth claims of those doctrines"?[33] It is worth noting that this inclusive "absolute necessity," however demanding, does not rise to the level of Fleck's constitutional principles of democratic deliberation. Ultimately Fleck's relatively weak positioning of inclusive diversity resonates with Daniels's placement of moral diversity: Both call for diversity to be respected in democratic deliberation, but neither makes it a core criterion for a fair decision-making process.

Both these accounts assume that deep moral commitments inevitably lead to irresolvable conflicts that are avoided by placing constraints on the processes of democratic deliberation. In both accounts, power, oppression, and privilege in social relations are only briefly acknowledged, usually in passing attention to marginalized and vulnerable social groups. But these relevant social relations seem to evaporate in the confidence that a fair process produces a level procedural playing field—as if deliberators could shed such differences and slip on a shroud of equity. On the whole, both theorists paint religious and cultural communities as the likely sources of inappropriate justifications for just health care decision making.

Segall embraces a luck egalitarian theory of justice in health and health care that holds the view that justice requires eliminating inequalities that result from bad luck.[34] Communities exist in two main ways in Segall's luck-sensitive framework: First, Segall attends to the political boundaries of a just health care system, explicitly affirming the nation-state, not communities, as the appropriate scope for health care justice. Second, justice requires distinguishing between health care needs and health care preferences, and Segall gives particular attention to defining the needs of religious and cultural communities.

In the name of distributive justice and intercommunal solidarity, Segall argues for a "unified" health care system in which all persons receive the same quality of care but in which the quantity and type of services depend of the aggregate needs of local communities. Correspondingly, he argues against the "devolution" of health services in which health care resources are distributed to "homogeneous" communities based on a per capita or equal-shares principle rather than on a more egalitarian, needs-based principle.[35] Such devolution he asserts is less egalitarian than a unified system and weakens social solidarity. It is unclear, first, why Segall assumes that communities are homogeneous, and second, why devolution requires an equal-shares rather than a needs-based distribution pattern. Without these assumptions his argument against devolution weakens considerably.

Interestingly, Segall limits his argument for unified health care systems to "functioning" plurinational societies.[36] Devolution in health care is allowed in societies that are irretrievably fragmented or where "one community is systematically discriminated against . . . in a way that cannot be repaired."[37] He likens devolution to divorce, "not something to be encouraged or actively sought" but allowable in extreme circumstances.[38] Segall contends that neither of his case-study countries, Belgium and Israel, are severely divided societies, and he does not offer an example of one. Ultimately it is unclear who decides whether a plurinational society is functioning and how that determination is made, as well as whether any extant society meets the threshold for a devolved health care system.

Segall contends that "the more accurate and authentic the perception of medical needs employed by the health care system in serving its population, the more just the health care system is."[39] This is a second significant way that communities, and specifically, community-related health care needs, inhabit this luck egalitarian theory. Segall is concerned to distinguish medical *needs* from medical *preferences* in cultural and religious communities, for at stake is the scope of responsibility for related health care.

Segall identifies four ways that membership in religious and cultural communities shape health care needs and preferences. If (1) cultural membership puts people at greater risk for ill health—his example is "alcohol abuse in a protestant society"[40]—or if (2) ill health produces a greater harm due to one's culture—for example, having a speech impediment in a culture that highly values speaking skills—then the health care needs that follow are legitimate and are rightly cared for in a just health care system. In contrast, (3) cultural nonmedical needs—such as male circumcision—are not considered legitimate health care needs because they do not involve a medical condition, even if a medical practitioner performs them. Similarly, (4) medical procedures and services that are more highly prized by specific cultures—for example, fetal screenings desired by cultures that emphasize "successful" children—are deemed medical "tastes" or preferences and are not legitimate medical needs in a just health care system.[41]

An important issue is who determines whether a claimed need is a legitimate need or a preference. Notably, members of a cultural community are not considered to be reliable and legitimate interpreters of their health care needs: "The relevant criterion for determining what counts as a need, then, is what an outside observer would identify as constituting a decent life in a certain community, and not (or not necessarily) what members of that community consider to constitute a decent life."[42] Thus religious and cultural communities are recognized as influential in shaping their members' health care needs and preferences but ultimately rejected as the legitimate definers of those needs in lieu of outsider interpretations of a decent community life. Resonant with the frameworks of Fleck and Daniels, this luck egalitarian account envisions religious and cultural communities as potentially threatening to a just, unified system of health care.

Across all three of these egalitarian theories of justice for health care—just health, just caring, and luck egalitarianism—subnational communities and their community members are depicted, in both subtle and explicit ways, as partial, unreasonable, discriminatory, irrelevant, unreliable, and undemocratic. In short, they are depicted as obstacles or threats to just decision-making processes.

Communities as Morally Inert

Capabilities approaches to justice in health care take a different course than egalitarian approaches by positing the fulfillment of human capabilities as the central aim of justice, rather than equality of opportunity or procedural fairness. As in the egalitarian frameworks, communities receive relatively minor attention. That said, the sort of attention they receive is typically different. In general, the capabilities approaches recognize individuals as community members, affirm the moral standing of individuals, and simultaneously deny that communities have moral standing. Rather than posit communities as a threat or obstacle to justice, communities tend to be relegated to the backseat of moral relevancy, rendering them, in effect, morally inert. Communities in Jennifer Ruger's health capability theory are largely implied, thus essentially invisible in relation to justice.[43] Communities are present but deemed morally immaterial in Sridhar Venkatapuram's health capability approach. And Madison Powers and Ruth Faden's theory of social justice both recognizes certain communities and rejects them as morally salient in relation to justice.[44]

Ruger grounds her health capability paradigm in a vision of human flourishing: "a view of society in which all people have the ability to realize central health capabilities—that is, to avoid premature death and escapable morbidity."[45] She argues that all persons "irrespective of class, gender, race, ethnicity,

or community" have a special obligation to provide these central health capabilities.[46] This representation of persons "irrespective" of particularity and of
community signals this framework's general eclipsing of communities.

Ruger mentions communities and groups occasionally in passing and often
by implication. For example, the universal responsibility to provide central
health capabilities is fulfilled, in Ruger's view, through shared health governance that is "shared among different individual and social structures, but with
the individual at the centre," and is "a continuum from individual to social
responsibility in which most cases lies somewhere along that continuum."[47]
Both these descriptions of responsibility for shared health governance imply
that there are morally relevant intermediary social structures, structures that
would reasonably include families and communities, though they are not
named as such. More directly, Ruger calls for "equipping individuals and communities" with needed resources for health capacity building but does not further develop this objective.[48]

At times, this health capability approach simply ignores communities and
social groups. For instance, Ruger applauds national social movements such as
feminist and civil rights movements for their contributions to changing communal values and norms regarding gender and racial equity. And she affirms
that social movements are vital to shifting present national norms and values to
those needed for future reforms in U.S. health policy.[49] Yet these social movements are presented as if they are devoid of actual communities—the racial,
cultural, gender, political, and religious communities that often create, support,
and maintain social movements. In effect, communities and their moral importance to social movements and to justice are invisible.

Relatedly, Ruger confirms cultural norms as powerful factors associated
with individual health agency, health, and justice. She highlights sub-Saharan
African "norms" of child rape, the subordination of women and persons with
AIDS, and disbelief in the sexual transmission of HIV, as well as U.S. norms
regarding substance use (adolescent drinking) and disability (autism).[50] But
these cultural norms are posited as the products of seemingly homogeneous
societies, not of particular cultural communities in particular social contexts,
thus again rendering invisible actual subnational communities.

At times Ruger briefly recognizes social groups or communities but then
explicitly or implicitly dismisses their moral relevance to health and social justice: "While group differences are important for policy and public health purposes, assessing individual disadvantage is the most morally relevant criterion
of justice."[51] In a generous reading, this passage allows that group disadvantage

might be considered a—but not the most—morally relevant criterion of justice, but this health capability paradigm does not address any such role for groups or communities.

Ruger is concerned that communitarian theories of justice like that of Walzer "allow the justification of health care to vary by community" and "taken to the extreme . . . could undermine political and social cooperation in societies that respect individual liberties and diversity."[52] This worry about social order and, by implication, conflict echoes the liberal egalitarian theories and suggests this concern as a possible source of Ruger's relative inattention to communities and groups. Though any view "taken to the extreme" is likely to be problematic, Ruger infers that community-based views of justice necessarily jeopardize health care justice.

In a second health capabilities theory, Venkatapuram advances a species-wide notion of health justice in which "every human being has a moral entitlement to a capability to be healthy . . . , and to a level that is commensurate with equal human dignity in the contemporary world."[53] He understands health capability to involve a universal and objective set of health goals, not community-specific health goals, and he locates universal entitlement to health capability in liberal social justice's "rock bottom" values of human freedom and "respect for the equal dignity" of all persons.[54]

Strongly critical of the individualism of the biomedical model, Venkatapuram supports the substantial findings of social epidemiology that identify close correlations between individuals, social groups, social conditions, and health. Despite his explicit acknowledgment that needless illness and premature death "heap on" particular social groups, Venkatapuram rejects the notion of group justice: "[Individuals who experience impairments and premature death] are not a distinct social class; impairments as well as mortality affect every human being over the lifespan."[55] In other words, all persons suffer disease and death; all persons do not constitute a discrete social group; and thus disproportionate disease burden is not a matter of group justice.

Venkatapuram acknowledges his "intuitive skepticism of giving groups ethical status, or rights to capabilities," and argues that the right to the capability to be healthy is an individual right,[56] although he seems to leave an opening: "Yet it is still uncertain whether inter-dependent individuals with shared ends constitute something more than just individuals. In any case, group level analysis of the CH [capability for health] is something that is aligned with the individual entitlement to the CH because it reflects the moral concern for individuals belonging to the groups."[57] In this view, individuals are group members; group membership may harm individual capability to be healthy, and therefore analyses of groups differences is in order; but in the end, group justice is deemed unsuitable to this understanding of health justice. Both Ruger's health capabilities paradigm and Venkatapuram's capability to be healthy theory recognize individuals as community or group members and individual health as related to group membership; they affirm a role for communities in health care, notably health promotion; and then they reject those communities as morally relevant to health justice.

Powers and Faden offer a theory of social justice that obligates societal institutions to provide the conditions for human well-being.[58] In this account, well-being is understood as being composed of six essential elements: health, personal security, reasoning, respect, attachment, and self-determination. Health encompasses the realms of public health, clinical medicine, and health policy, and it is in relation to public health that their primary attention to groups and communities is found. Powers and Faden distinguish two "points" or aims of social justice. One is an aspirational or positive point requiring the improvement of the health of all; the other is a remedial or negative point requiring "policing" and "aggressive public health intervention" to identify "densely woven patterns of disadvantage" that produce health inequalities and limit well-being.[59] They recognize health disparities between "socially dominant groups" and "socially disadvantaged groups" and declare that the "patterns of systematic disadvantage linked to group membership are among the most invidious, thoroughgoing, and difficult to escape."[60]

Powers and Faden explicitly affirm that "groups matter" in public health and in social justice—more specifically, the relatively poor health of members of socially disadvantaged groups matters when health inequalities are tied to group membership.[61] Women, African Americans, and persons living in poverty all represent disadvantaged groups with morally troubling health statuses related to systemic group oppression. That said, and echoing the perspectives of Ruger and Venkatapuram, groups are morally important as aggregates of individuals, but they have no little or no moral import as groups per se. About this Powers and Faden are clear: "For public health and health policy generally, groups matter, but we are not interested in the health, other dimensions of well-being, or rights of groups per se. Rather, our focus on groups is contingent on what we understand to be true of how the world works. That is, we are interested in the well-being, flourishing, and rights of individuals, but in the real, historically situated world, how individuals fare is generally a function of the status, standing, and position within densely woven patterns of systemic disadvantage of the groups of which they are a part."[62]

Notably, groups in this theory of social justice are primarily associated with the negative, corrective point of justice: Socially disadvantaged groups are the objects of public health's remedial work. Socially dominant groups appear minimally and usually in contrast to socially dominated groups, bringing health inequalities into sharp relief. Despite Powers and Faden's recognition of group disadvantage, groups matter to the extent that their disadvantage impedes individual health; groups are not active participants in determining the nature of health, well-being, or social justice.

Identifying communities and their moral roles in these six justice frameworks reveals significant yet often neglected features of contemporary health care justice discourse. As noted, health care justice theories have little room for communities, conceiving the ones they do address as either morally inert or as obstacles to health care justice.[63] Consistent with the egalitarian justice theories examined earlier in this chapter, the central moral actors in capability theories are nation-states and individuals. In general contrast to the egalitarian theories, capability theories recognize groups and communities as influential to individual health and health care and, at the same time, reject their moral pull on justice in health care.

Some of these theories take seriously the fact that particular communities are significant meaning makers. Religious and cultural communities often embrace comprehensive worldviews that encompass deeply held norms and values related to health and health care. It is precisely the powerful meaning making that occurs in some communities that leads these theorists to perceive these communities as obstacles or threats. In Daniels's processes of democratic deliberation, for example, cultural and religious perspectives are "unreasonable" owing to their inaccessibility to nonbelievers. Similarly, Fleck's democratic deliberation requires deliberators to give public reasons unrelated to their deep religious or philosophic views because, in his view, only such public reasons serve the public interest, liberal neutrality, and respect for all persons. Segall acknowledges the culturally specific health care needs and preferences of cultural communities but privileges outsiders as better able to identify community needs.

Groups and communities bound by social class, gender, and race are typically considered vulnerable and disadvantaged subjects of social inequities as well as of inequities in health status and health care services. Implied in this characterization of communities is a recognition that communities and their social relations shape individual health and health care—two of the community dimensions of health and health care described in chapter 1. Powers and

Faden, for example, primarily address groups that are subject to "densely woven patterns of disadvantage." To the degree that these groups experience systemic disadvantage and oppression, Powers and Faden argue that it is public health's responsibility to monitor these groups in order to "police" that disadvantage, and as such, these groups and communities become sites of intervention in the name of individual health and well-being.[64]

Notably, socially advantaged or dominant groups (per Powers and Faden) and better-off groups (per Daniels) receive the barest attention, but by implication these groups appear to be white, male, middle income (or higher), with relatively good health status and access to health care. This selective and disproportionate attention to disadvantaged groups illustrates Karla Holloway's observation of bioethics, in which people of color and women are more prominently represented as community members and as the *public* than are dominant persons, especially those who are white and men, who are more typically portrayed as private individuals.[65] The moral and social relationships of power, oppression, and privilege between disadvantaged and advantaged groups remain largely unexamined in these theories.

It is striking to notice how marginalized communities are *not* represented in this justice discourse. Communities are not cast as heterogeneous and dynamic entities, composed of morally authoritative community members who participate in just health care decision making. The recognized communities do not participate in creating and supporting the central moral values critical to these theories or frameworks. Ruger's model of shared health governance, for example, asserts that multilevel social structures, ostensibly including communities, have responsibility for creating the conditions for health capability but also does not speak directly of those communities and their responsibilities. Daniels asserts that health is morally important owing to its effects on life opportunities and that the American value of equal opportunity "reflects people's real interests." Yet this understanding of health itself is not the outcome of just democratic deliberative processes vetted by accountability for reasonableness criteria. The various moral understandings of health and health care espoused by diverse communities have little to no place in these theories.

Furthermore, some of these theorists assert that their national—in other words, subglobal—conceptions of health care justice are important to understanding global health justice. Yet, paradoxically, they reject the notion that subnational conceptions of health justice are important to understanding national or societal health care justice.

On the whole, these health care justice theories have limited engagement with the range of communities and community relations most central to health and health care. What we need is a theory of health care justice that recognizes multiple and diverse communities with their particular values and under-standings as relevant health and health care. Ultimately we need a theory that engages heterogeneous communities as substantive contributors to the creation of health care justice.

Chapter 3

Communities Constrained

A Liberal Communitarian View

Not all theories of health justice neglect communities or understand them as impediments to justice. Ezekiel Emanuel's liberal communitarian vision of health justice, for example, places multiple and diverse communities at the center of just health care.[1] Justice, says Emanuel, is the fair allocation of medical care services guided by a community's conception of the good life, that is, by the community's "accepted moral ideals, traditions and customs, accepted practices, and paradigmatic precedents of history, that is, stories."[2] In this vision, different communities are constituted by different conceptions of the good life, and all communities commit to democratic deliberation as the means of negotiating their conception of the good life and its implications for health care. This chapter provides a close examination of this community-centered vision, revealing its strengths and limits and, along with chapter 2, helps us to identify the significant features of an alternate notion of justice in health care.

Applying his model of deliberative community to health care, Emanuel envisions dividing the United States into roughly ten thousand communities, each with approximately twenty-five thousand members sharing a particular conception of the good life. Each community would establish a community health program (CHP) to organize the delivery of health care services to its members. Drawing on its particular conception of the good life, each community would deliberate to determine and prioritize the services offered, as well as to formulate specific—particularly ethical—policies related to the allocation of resources.

Community health programs would be federated into a national system overseen by federal and state regulatory boards. These boards would make sure that every citizen is a CHP member, monitor for discrimination and other rights violations in enrollment and participation practices, and mediate conflicts among CHPs as well as between CHPs and other health care institutions. Each CHP would employ or contract with physicians, hospitals, and other providers to provide health care services to its members. Community health programs would receive annual capitated payments from member vouchers drawn from a centralized federal health care trust fund into which all current health care expenditures (including those for public programs like Medicare and Medicaid, private health plan premiums, and direct patient payments) would be collected and pooled. The federal board would distribute vouchers worth five years of payments to each person (or family), and some funds would be set aside at the federal level for health research. Individual CHPs could decide to spend more or less per capita on health care—for example, by instituting an additional self-tax or by cashing in part or all of its government vouchers.

Emanuel outlines three levels of distributive justice in health care: political, medical, and patient centered. At the political level—that is, the societal or national level—decisions are made about how much of society's financial resources should be devoted to medicine. At the patient-centered level, decisions are made about which individual patients will receive specific, often scarce, services. Emanuel's vision focuses on the *medical* level, where decisions are made about which medical services a CHP should offer. The identification and ranking of guaranteed medical services requires the principled negotiation of concerns at both the political and the patient-centered levels—including the articulation of ethical ideals, typically embedded in a community's conception of the good life. The labeling of the intermediary level as "medical" implicitly restricts the scope of health care to medical care. This is curious given that decision making at this level is done, in theory, by communities and not by physicians.

Emanuel proposes a vision in which communities with very different conceptions of the good life have the opportunity to embody their specific conceptions in the health care they receive and pay for. Given its particular conception, one CHP might offer a wide array of preventive and primary-care services but not organ transplants, whereas another CHP, based on its own conception, might offer extensive tertiary care, including organ transplants but few preventive services. Notably, this differentiated provision of health care services would not be unjust, according to Emanuel, because "justice is not realized by comparing entitlements to individual services, but by respecting the community's particular conception of the good life expressed in its distribution of goods."[3] Each community determines the normative standards of justice to which its members agree and by which they are bound, based on that community's conception of the good life. Accordingly, there is no single standard of justice for U.S. health care based on a common conception of the good life.

However, Emanuel does not leave justice entirely to community determination. He asserts an overarching national principle of justice: the principle of equal access where, "within any particular political community, all citizens should be treated equally and should be entitled to access to the same basic medical services as determined by that polity's conception of the good life."[4] Community health programs with conceptions of the good life that affirm unequal access for some of its members are prohibited. Thus, this national standard of equal access serves to both trump and complement the community standard. Emanuel justifies this principle of equal access by recognizing it as a "strong" and "settled intuition" that "strikes a deep resonance within American culture."[5] Three elements of health care justice deserve special scrutiny given their centrality to Emanuel's vision: justice, community, and deliberation.

Justice as Equal Access to CHP-Determined Medical Care Services

With this two-part notion of justice—justice as (a) equal access to (b) CHP-determined medical care services—Emanuel expands liberal notions of justice. In his theory, justice includes democratic political participation (regarding conceptions of the good life) *within* CHPs—that is, within subnational communities. Accordingly, justice requires that "the citizens of a particular CHP are guaranteed those services that fulfill their avowed conception of the good life,"[6] in which a citizen is defined as "a potential participant in democratic deliberations."[7]

This understanding of just health care is both well steeped in the classic liberal distributive paradigm of justice and a sophisticated effort to move beyond it. It is distributive in its fundamental orientation to two end-state patterns of distribution: (1) the universal CHP membership required by the principle of equal access, and (2) the community-specific patterns of distribution of medical care services. As a "settled intuition," equal access is a nondeliberated, nonnegotiable pattern of distribution, whereas the patterns of community-specific distribution of medical care services are born of deliberation and negotiation.

Emanuel's concern for the political processes related to justice—that is, to the social creation, refinement, and embodiment of conceptions of the good life through deliberation—introduces an important relational dimension to his distributive framework. Here communities are understood as the creators, not simply the bearers of social goods and of justice. Persons with sufficiently similar conceptions of the good life join together to form a health care community and create community-based health care policy that reflects their particular conception of the good life. They understand "just health care" to mean equal access to a community-designed set of services and policies. As such, in Emanuel's vision, subnational communities play a central role in the creation of justice in health care.

However, three characteristics of this view of justice seriously constrain it: its narrow scope of community-defined justice, its assumption of health care services as commodity-like rather than as relational and inevitably imbued with power relations, and its medical and biomedical biases. First, communities' conceptions of the good life and community decision making are introduced only *after* justice has been confined to the tasks of ranking and selecting medical services. This restriction means that conceptions of the good life are allowed to inform only distributive issues of justice in health care; nondistributive issues—for example, the relative authority of CHPs and physicians—are preempted.

Second, each CHP designs a unique package of services. It does this through a process of weighing and balancing, ranking and selecting many services that are then purchased with vouchers and dispersed as needed. Neglected in this somewhat commodified view of health care are its relational dimensions, especially as they relate to *interpersonal* care. Emanuel speaks little of the caring aspects of health care, though he does attend briefly to the physician-patient relationship, which he suggests can be a friendship: "[This liberal communitarian proposal] should be seen as an attempt to minimize the economic and merely technical aspects of the physician-patient relationship by reclaiming the traits that make this a relationship between friends, albeit friends who have differences of knowledge, need, and vulnerability. By stressing the practice of medicine as an enterprise suffused with moral deliberation, this work should provide a justification for preserving and enriching the best aspects of the traditional physician-patient relationship so threatened by contemporary circumstances."[8]

In this passage, intricate inequities become simple "differences"; Emanuel ignores the complexities of social and power relations between patients and physicians as well as their implications for just health care. Moreover, he fails to address other caring relationships, such as those between patients and other care givers, and those between care givers—professional or otherwise.

Ultimately, this invocation of interpersonal deliberation confuses Emanuel's overall focus on the communal deliberation and articulation of worthy ideals.

Finally, medicine, medical ethics, and physicians are Emanuel's near-exclusive concern. This strong medical orientation is amply evident in his medicalized notion of health care, his labeling of the community level of distribution as the "medical level" and of this overall project as "medical ethics," and the consistent priority given to physicians as health care professionals. Furthermore, this vision assumes that communities embrace only a Western, biomedical model of health and disease. Despite Emanuel's inclusion of a wide range of conceptions of the good life, he ignores nonbiomedical frameworks of health and healing. Particular communities' conceptions of the good life might quite reasonably lead to religious and cultural beliefs and practices including complementary and alternative medicine as their chosen health care modalities, even alongside biomedicine. Together, the limited decision-making role that Emanuel sees for communities, combined with his misleading view of health care as a package of discrete and commodified medical services, portends problems for the clear conceptualization and effective expression of justice in health care.

Communities Bound by Conceptions of the Good Life

Emanuel's hypothetical and self-defining political communities are each bound by a shared conception of the good life that, in turn, shapes a particular CHP. He specifically identifies diverse communities and CHPs, including Orthodox Jewish, democratic individualist, lesbian, Amish, American Indian, Mormon, fundamentalist Protestant, extreme free market, elderly, homosexual, white, Hispanic, the Adam Smith CHP, the Jeremy Bentham CHP, and the Moral Majority CHP. Emanuel also refers, though confusingly, to both employment-based communities and geographic communities. He references "work-site CHPs" despite the improbability that upward of twenty-five thousand employees of the same company would share the same conception of the good life and despite his desire to disconnect access to health care from employment.[9] Emanuel consistently presumes a geographic dimension of many communities in his frequent references to them as "local" and in his promotion of "local control" of health care policies.[10] Yet he explicitly dismisses geography as a basis for community, doubting the possibility of a shared social life in neighborhoods: "Contemporary neighborhoods tend not to reflect any shared religious, cultural, or philosophical conceptions among the residents. Indeed, probably the only shared traits among neighborhood residents are socioeconomic class, income, and wealth."[11] These assertions are dubious given the communal social life that socioeconomic class frequently entails, not to mention the relative racial and cultural—and not simply income homogeneity—of many U.S. neighborhoods.

In elaborating the sources of conceptions of the good life, Emanuel declares, "An individual is born into a social world and inherits a tradition and a past that he [*sic*] has neither chosen nor created."[12] This understanding of the person as born into *a single* tradition does not admit the possibility that persons inherit multiple morally informative traditions and communities and thus may have multiple, even conflicting, sources for a conception of the good life. The idea that persons not only might be born into multiple traditions and communities but also might choose to belong to and to participate in more than one community is also alien to this liberal communitarian vision.

In Emanuel's vision, not all conceptions of the good life are permissible. All CHP conceptions of the good life must include a commitment to deliberative democracy; Emanuel vacillates on whether and how nondeliberative conceptions of the good life would be excluded. For example, Jeremy Bentham CHPs—understood as strictly utilitarian and without a commitment to deliberation—"would be permitted within the liberal communitarian vision, [though] their proliferation would undermine the stability of the vision."[13] It is unclear whose responsibility it is to prevent the initial formation and funding of nondeliberative CHPs.

Moreover, "unfairly" discriminatory conceptions of the good life also violate the spirit of democratic deliberation and are not allowed in this liberal communitarian vision. Emanuel explains:

> There is a difference between communities that espouse a conception of the good life, excluding those who do not similarly espouse the ideal, and communities that espouse a conception of the good life in which the ideal is exclusion. The difference is between a conception of the good life with an internal, positive ideal and a conception of the good life based on the opposition to and denigration of others. While the first view will oppose some conceptions of the good life, it has its own ideals that can be characterized without counter-defining them against the ideals of others. The content of the second is provided only in opposition to others. This second form becomes discriminatory when it aims not merely at separation but at denigration and domination of the groups it opposes. In its discriminatory form it conflicts with the respect for the freedom and equality of citizens that is essential for deliberation.

Without commitment to this respect, there is no chance of realizing the liberal communitarian vision or any democratic political vision.[14]

Conceptually, as well as in practice, this distinction between conceptions is strained. Emanuel recognizes that positive ideals are, by definition, opposed to other ideals, but he does not offer an example of a conception that exists "only in opposition to others."

Conceptions of the good life range widely in their degree of structure and development. Some conceptions are well formed and detailed, others are more of an "outline," and still others are even less defined: "We can expect that many CHPs will form among people who share some specific views on a handful of the most visible and controversial medical ethical issues, but have not explored other issues or elaborated more abstract moral positions. . . . This process of deliberation would be more one of creating collective values than of interpreting existing ones."[15]

These weaker conceptions of the good life are problematic to this liberal communitarian vision because communities are, by definition, bound by identifiable and articulated conceptions of the good life. Are vague or shallow conceptions of the good life sufficient foundation for the formation of communities, the establishment of CHPs, and the determination of justice? Without a strong and clear conception of the good life, why would these communities form, and why should they be entrusted with the determination of justice? Granted that traditions and conceptions of the good life are subject to ongoing deliberation, how much of a conception is necessary to bind a community? A CHP? Justice? Emanuel seems to presume that even weak conceptions of the good life are sufficiently binding and thus does not address these questions.

Emanuel's tendency toward reduction and singularity is also evident in his assertion that some traditions, communities, and CHPs embrace a unified set of beliefs and practices:

> In some communities the outlines of this shared vision [the conception of the good life] would be obvious. All members would recognize the same articulation of the vision, and indeed this commonality would be what has brought them together. This would be most characteristic of a religious community, such as a Mormon or a fundamentalist Protestant community, that has a shared tradition, canonical texts, recognized authority figures, fairly detailed views of acceptable medical practices, and possibly already existing hospitals that operate according to its views. But this might also be true of communities that share a well-developed secular philosophy.[16]

That these are relatively agreeable and cohesive communities is also implied in Emanuel's sweeping and frequently stereotypic descriptions of CHPs and their conceptions of the good life. To quote just three examples: "An elderly community might . . . fund all life-saving treatments but leav[e] the cost of nursing home care and medical devices to individuals";[17] "A homosexual CHP might . . . decide to allocate its resources to out-patient drug treatments for AIDS patients aimed at forestalling life-threatening infections and tumors, but might decide that in-hospital life-saving treatments should not receive funding while hospice care would be supplied";[18] and "A lesbian community with a shared view of feminism might want to limit its members to fellow lesbians."[19]

Whereas Emanuel minimizes differences within communities, he maximizes differences between them. He finds each conception of the good life to be so unique as to be incommensurable with one another, and thus he rejects the notion that one "compromise" plan for a nationwide medical system could be devised.[20] This adamant claim about the incommensurability of conceptions of the good life is surprising given Emanuel's point that different communities will undoubtedly share some elements of conceptions of the good life. Furthermore, this vision assumes at least two important national agreements or compromises found in Emanuel's triple-level scheme of distribution involving the political, medical, and patient-centered levels of health care. Recall that the determination of justice at the medical level requires the balancing of resource limits at the political level and the principle of equal access at the patient-centered level. Emanuel assumes national agreement both on the portion of the federal budget dedicated to health care and on the principle of equal access. These agreements imply some level of compatibility among conceptions of the good life and serve as evidence that important distributive decisions are possible at the national level. As noted above, Emanuel does not discuss the place or function of conceptions of the good life at either the political or patient-centered levels; he focuses exclusively on the medical level.

All persons are guaranteed membership in some CHP, though not in a particular CHP. Once admitted to a CHP, a person can chose to leave and join another CHP but that person cannot be expelled by the community. Notably, this potential fluidity of communities could undermine this vision's need for sustained deliberation. In addition, significant tensions may surround CHP admission and membership. Emanuel presumes that persons have a choice among CHPs, yet two elements of this vision mitigate against this choice: (1) CHPs are characterized by particular conceptions of the good life, and there is no guarantee that multiple compatible CHPs exist where one lives; and (2)

CHPs admit candidates for membership based on a CHP judgment about a candidate's commitment to that CHP's conception of the good life: "Each communal polity will be limited in size, and the members of the community will have to decide who are its members and who are not."[21]

In this vision, community members and member candidates must have "some commitment to recognizing, elaborating, affirming, and abiding by the community's particular conception of the good life."[22] Immediately, two questions arise: (1) What is the community's particular conception of the good life? (2) And what does it mean to recognize, elaborate, affirm, and abide by it? In terms of the second question, this kind of commitment to a particular conception of the good life would be rather difficult to make since, as suggested already, such conceptions may not be well defined and articulated.

Emanuel allows discrimination in membership if it is deemed "necessary to sustain a community's commitment to a particular conception of the good life." He elaborates his understanding of legitimate exclusion through an analogy with nonbelievers attending a religious service:

> Having non-believing members of a community is analogous to having silent considerate non-participants in a religious service. They do not overtly disturb or interrupt the religious service. Nevertheless, because their presence does not contribute to it, they "flatten" the religious service by creating a dead space and thereby detract from it. Similarly, nonbelieving members do not perpetuate the community's traditions; they do not articulate and specify the community's ideals; they do not sustain the community's activities. The non-contribution to the community's distinctive character is not benign but a detraction. For this reason many communities may not want to accept such respectful but non-believing people as members. The exclusion of respectful non-believers is necessary to sustain communities. This is a position the liberal communitarian vision should endorse even when it means that the communities may exclude individuals from membership on the basis of age, sex, religion, and the like.[23]

Emanuel's strong penchant for sameness and conflict avoidance is strikingly revealed in his representation of nonmember presence as "a dead space," a "detraction," and a "noncontribution." Decisions about whether particular beliefs constitute a commitment to, or a detraction from, a conception of the good life are highly subjective; state health oversight boards are primarily responsible to assure that CHP applicants are not unfairly discriminated against. However, Emanuel notes that, because many states have a history of discrimination, it may be beneficial for them to have federal oversight and guidelines on membership and participation.[24] Thus, presumably, nonmembers will participate in adjudicating whether a community's conception of the good life matches its actions and behaviors (resounding with Shlomi Segall's notion of community outsiders as adjudicators of community needs; see chapter 2).

To recap, the "good-life" communities of this liberal communitarian vision are multiple, deliberative, and nongeographic communities that share a relatively homogeneous, often weak, and always incommensurable conception of the good life. This notion of what is essentially a political community undermines Emanuel's theory of justice in several ways. Recall that Emanuel's idea of justice requires that a community deliberate to determine its shared conception of the good life and attendant health care policies. In his theory, communal deliberation is the fundamental activity of communities in their efforts (*a*) to form and develop conceptions of the good life and (*b*) to make distributive decisions and policies at the medical level. Yet how much deliberation will occur in communities that, by definition, share fundamental ideals? How much deliberation can take place in nongeographic communities? A closer look at this deliberative role in the next section reveals additional and important limits of this vision.

Community Deliberation

Emanuel's communities are meaning makers in that they create, deliberate, and refine their group values, including community-specific meanings of justice and health care. Given that communities are defined by an agreed-upon conception of the good life, it seems that these groups would experience relatively little serious conflict. Emanuel understands any conflict to be either resolvable when it does not threaten members' commitment to a community or fundamental when it destabilizes the community's shared commitment to its conception of the good life. Emanuel illustrates the distinction between resolvable and fundamental conflicts with the case of Orthodox Jews and the issues of brain death and the harvesting of organs for transplantation: "As long as those debating appeal to recognized authorities, traditions, and texts, Halakah, but disagree over their interpretation and specification, there is a resolvable conflict. If the conflict arises because one participant questions the authority of Halakah, then there is a fundamental conflict. In this way, resolvable conflicts are inherent and integral to deliberative democracy, the basis of deliberations. But no political community can withstand persistent fundamental disagreements."[25]

Yet it is not obvious that the questioning of a tradition's authorities constitutes "no common commitment" or necessarily threatens a community's very existence. In fact, different interpretations often rest on different understandings of authority. This dichotomous view of conflict distorts the deliberative process, functioning to reduce diversity and affirm uniformity.

But for Emanuel, the consequences of attempting to blend incommensurable conceptions of the good life within a single community would entail offense and "less deliberation and more conflict": "Using geography as a basis for CHPs will force people who espouse incommensurable conceptions of the good life to deliberate and formulate policies. Inevitably the policies will offend individuals whose conceptions of the good life conflict with the policies. And if the conceptions of the good life are truly incommensurable, then we should not expect compromise positions. The inevitable result will be less deliberation and more conflict resolved only by ballot box power."[26] However, it is unavoidable that democratic deliberation requires difference and thus conflict. Even Emanuel notes that public participation entails "argument and persuasion."[27]

Emanuel foresees that many of us will choose not to participate in deliberations, though he finds "natural incentives and interests" to do so, such as our personal needs for services and growing public concern about medical ethical issues. In Emanuel's view, participation by CHP members "depends upon citizens' viewing moments of participation both as meaningful aspects of their self-conception and as practically effective. . . . Consequently, the extent of participation in CHPs depends upon the suitability of structures for this participation, the commitment of CHPs and their leading members to foster such democratic discussions, and the efficacy of such deliberations in shaping CHP policies. With institutions promoting meaningful and effective communal deliberations, citizens will tend to view participation as a part of their lives."[28] In order to discern the necessary features of communal deliberation and their role in shaping just health care, I examine in depth each of Emanuel's three determinants of participation: the suitability of structures for participation, the commitment of CHPs and their leading members to foster democratic discussions, and the efficacy of deliberations in shaping CHP policies.

Suitable Structures for Participation

Emanuel attributes the contemporary lack of communal deliberation in health care to health care's privatization, organizational bureaucracy, and financing mechanisms. His proposed financing and administrative structures—a centralized health care trust fund and CHPs bound by shared conceptions of the good life—are designed, in part, to enable a stable pool of patients to engage in democratic deliberations about fundamental values and specific policies over a sustained period. He suggests incentivizing participation, for example, by having employers give employees time away from work for their involvement. Despite Emanuel's dismissal of geographic communities as the bases of CHPs, the deliberation he envisions occurs in various forms requiring interpersonal and institutional proximity, from town meetings of the whole community debating a wide range of issues, to appointed committees addressing specific issues.

While Emanuel says little about power in democratic deliberations, he acknowledges the hierarchical nature of current decision making in health care institutions and affirms the democratic nature of his proposed deliberations. He contends that "the institutional structures necessary for deliberative democracy are neither obvious nor extant; they must be imagined and specified."[29] That said, Emanuel also predicts that "the deliberation on and formulations of CHP medical policies would not be very different from the types of deliberations that currently occur at many HMOs and hospitals that require their own policies. . . . The substantive difference between existing deliberations and those imagined here is in the parties to the deliberations."[30]

This "add citizens and stir" model of deliberation raises the question of how much genuine authority or power CHP members would have in democratic deliberation. Citing various deliberative mechanisms used by the members of the Group Health Cooperative of Puget Sound (a health maintenance organization, or HMO), Emanuel concedes that, although HMO members can "discuss critical issues" and make "resolutions," they do not have policy-making power.[31] This participation hardly meets Emanuel's own democratic deliberative goal of "having citizens decide what laws, policies, and social conditions will govern their lives."[32] Yet, despite the virtual absence of this sort of communal deliberation in most HMOs, Emanuel frequently compares CHPs to HMOs.[33]

Structures that enable true democratic deliberation are needed not only for deliberations within a CHP but also for deliberation among CHPs and with other local institutions. Emanuel acknowledges that interactions between local CHPs and with other social institutions could strengthen both health care services and local political structures for everyone. Community health programs would interact also at the state, regional, and national levels, as necessary, to deal with issues resolvable only at those levels. Presumably, individual CHPs' particular conceptions of the good life would be brought to bear on all levels of decision making; for this reason alone, it is unclear how CHPs would, or even could, work together if, according to Emanuel, they (a) hold incommensurable conceptions of the good life and (b) are nongeographic in nature.

Community Health Program Member Commitment
to Foster Democratic Discussions

Community health programs, by definition, have a basic commitment to democratic deliberation. As noted, Emanuel recognizes the hierarchical nature of current health care decision making as a barrier to democratic deliberations and associates this problem with bureaucratic and financial structures. Although he also acknowledges the unequal nature of the physician-patient relationship, he ignores its traditionally nondemocratic effects, especially as they relate to organized medicine. Only in passing does he acknowledge the obstructionist role that the medical profession has historically played with regard to communal deliberation.

Historically, neighborhood health centers, prepaid group health plans, and medical cooperatives were met with active medical opposition, both local and national. Though Emanuel attempts to align these health care institutions and their communal forms of deliberation with his liberal communitarian vision, he fails to recognize that these institutions were established, and have survived, on the margins of traditional medicine and, ultimately, despite its resistance. Rather, Emanuel blames the federal government for the "failure" of community health centers and, thus, of communal deliberation: "If there is any reason for the failure of these centers, it is less intrinsic than a consequence of the constantly changing policies from Washington and ultimately their abandonment by the federal government."[34] Given Emanuel's strong bias in favor of the medical establishment, his dismissal of that establishment from significant responsibility for the current scarcity of communal deliberation is particularly problematic.

About CHP deliberations, Emanuel asserts that doctors are not only the "guardians of medical ethical issues" but also agents of the community in that arena; for that reason, their opinions "should carry significant influence."[35] Here he attempts to distinguish the realms of physician and community authority: Physicians should determine medical and professional standards, which include criteria for what treatments to offer to which tests to conduct. Communal decisions, that is, those appropriate to all citizen-members including physician citizen-members, include "ethical policies, defining priorities among services, establishing guidelines for the treatment of incompetent patients, outlining the type of informed consent procedures to be instituted, and the like."[36]

In practice, these realms of decision making are not rigidly separable. Many issues require integrated decision making—for example, the medical selection of the most appropriate therapies necessarily is intertwined with the communal determination concerning the priority of services.

We may also reasonably question Emanuel's commitment to democratic decision making in light of certain claims he makes. For example: "CHPs would constitute an alternative more hospitable both to facilitating communal input on those matters where communal values are determinative and retaining professional control over those policy matters where standards are properly defined by physicians. As such, CHPs should constitute an important institutional arrangement that unites democratic deliberations with professional autonomy."[37] This wording is telling: Communities have "input" while professionals have "control" in their respective realms of decision making, and, more important, Emanuel posits professional authority as distinct from democratic deliberations rather than as a part of it.

In yet another revealing claim, Emanuel states that "medicine should be viewed more as a unique moral enterprise engaging us—both physicians and patients—in interpreting our shared values for guidance concerning the needs of life. Among the normal circumstances of life, it is *only in the practice of medicine* that we are required to confront the meaning of human frailty and finitude and the many entwined ethical questions."[38] With less-than-subtle medical hubris, Emanuel discounts life's myriad experiences of human frailty and finitude and privileges those associated with the practice of medicine. Likewise, his book on liberal communitarianism for health care is titled *The Ends of Human Life: Medical Ethics in a Liberal Polity.*

The limited scope and authority of communal deliberation is also evident in Emanuel's description of the possible tasks of a CHP committee on the physician-patient relationship. This committee's role would be to "consider" various possible consent forms or even to design treatment forms; they could also "consider" ways to store and secure patient records, including issues involving access to those records.[39] While the design of forms and records storage are important issues, a committee on the physician-patient relationship could deliberate far more substantial concerns, for example, the issue at hand—the relative scope of physician and citizen authority and responsibility—or the nature of physician-patient "friendship." Once again, Emanuel has narrowed the scope of communal decision making. Yet in seeming contradiction to this, he simultaneously asserts the need to broaden the subjects of discussion, since "the more significant the decision, the greater will be the interest in participation."[40]

As Emanuel contends, truly democratic deliberations will require considerable institutional change. However, while proposing radical changes in financing and administration, he leaves the profession of medicine essentially unexamined and untouched. He does call for physicians "to begin developing the institutional structures necessary for increased democratic deliberations on medical ethical questions," but he offers little substantive analysis or advice regarding the professional barriers to such change.[41]

The Efficacy of Deliberations in Shaping CHP Policies

This liberal communitarian vision clearly assumes that citizen deliberation, based on conceptions of the good life, can effectively shape specific institutional policies. Emanuel recognizes that these new communal deliberations will be relatively inefficient by conventional standards. Indeed, he casts a rather negative light on citizen participation: "The process of deliberations and policy formation will be longer and more clumsy than it is currently. Indeed, many of the CHP members may lack information or have faulty information on relevant issues; they may be relatively inarticulate; they may be impassioned about minor issues; they may lack the knowledge or skills to develop coherent policies."[42] While all this may be the case, this characterization implies that these inefficiencies are somehow peculiar to citizens and do not exist, as well, among administrators and physicians. The actual efficacy of communal deliberations in shaping CHP policy is unknown and will depend greatly upon the institutionalized structures of participation.

One goal of the liberal communitarian ideal is "to make the entire range of policies cohere within a single conception of the good life."[43] Though achieving some level of coherence between ethical values and policies is a reasonable possibility, it seems unlikely that all of the necessary CHP policies can meaningfully cohere within one, often weakly articulated, conception of the good life. Emanuel does not offer additional standards for the efficacy of deliberation.

On the whole, Emanuel's liberal communitarian vision offers a sophisticated and constructive attempt to embody community-based ethical values in norms of justice for health care and real-world health care practices. His conception of community justice draws on national and community sources, though it is largely discerned through community-based democratic deliberation. In this, he goes further in understanding the importance of communities in any discussion of health care, and in allowing communities a role in health care justice, than most theorists of just health care, including those discussed in chapter 2. However, the deliberation central to Emanuel's vision is constrained by (*a*) its restriction to a narrow range of medicalized distributive decisions; (*b*) the romantic view of communities as independent, nongeographic groups sharing internally homogeneous, though externally incommensurable, conceptions of the good life, and providing little ground for democratic deliberation; and (*c*) the lack of participatory structures to ensure meaningful community member deliberation and decision making.

What we need is an understanding of community justice for health care that includes diversely constituted communities—not only those bound by agreement to a particular conception of the good life. Such an understanding must address community membership criteria issues, attend to power relations and participatory structures within and among communities, and recognize communities as social institutions that exist in relation to, and often in tension with, other social institutions, such as the nation-state.

Chapter 4

Community Justice

We *can* risk considering seriously the meaning the other gives to the world; building communities of support that have openness to the other at the center of their strength; surrendering our tendencies to omniscience without surrendering to despair; learning the particular content of just and fitting care.

—Margaret Farley

A common starting point for considerations of justice in health care is a narrative about an individual's experiences of health care injustice. As such, it would be fitting to begin this chapter about community justice in health care with a story about injustices related to a person's belonging to a particular community or group. The challenge is how to choose one among the many: Stories of being denied access to health care or to optimal health care because one is "of color"—African American, Latin@, Asian American, indigenous, or more—or because one is low income; uninsured; undocumented; pregnant; lesbian, gay, bisexual, trans, or queer (LGBTQ); a woman; disabled; imprisoned; seriously ill. Stories of living in physical, social, and economic conditions that make individual, family, and community health difficult, if not impossible. Stories of speaking out about one's needs, one's community or communities' needs, and encountering silence, indifference, or disrespect. Stories of loved ones or strangers who died preventable deaths, who live with preventable chronic illness, and those who will die of both. And then there are stories in the language of social epidemiology: Stories of mortality, morbidity, and disability rates stratified by income, race, ethnicity, and gender. Stories that are not randomly or equitably distributed. Stories that are not only past but painfully present. Forming health care communities where all these stories can be spoken, be heard, and be seriously engaged and where the meanings and practices of just health care are created is the work of community justice.

Just health care in the United States is surely "justice in the making"[1]—a vision, an aspiration, or—as Ezekiel Emanuel notes in his liberal-communitarian framework—"a reconstructive ideal."[2] Visions are necessary, for as Beverly Harrison reminds us, "People must have hope that something more than the present order of things is possible if they are to act together in the face of dehumanizing power."[3] And visions are powerful. In exploring Martin Luther King Jr.'s vision of the Beloved Community, Bryan N. Massingale echoes Harrison: "Visions illumine possibilities that are overlooked, paths not taken, potentials that lie dormant, and capacities not yet developed."[4] For Massingale a vision is also a "passion [that] can lead to and ground effective justice praxis" and "has the power to transform even recalcitrant realities."[5] Visions are also "reflexive" in that they will be reshaped over time as social conditions change and as more and different persons participate in the envisioning and praxis of justice.[6]

Community justice is one such vision of just health care in the making. Community justice is a vision of health care organized to respect the health-related meanings and values of multiple and diverse communities by coming to a set of agreed to—and in this sense, shared—meanings and values that guide the community's decision making about health care. Community justice is a moral vision that sets out three normative justice criteria at the community level regarding the requisite features of community, of care, and of community member participation. Before delving into this vision, I explore the underlying ethical grounding of community justice, that is, the obligation to respect persons as individuals who are also community members.

Justice and Respect for Persons as Community Members

"We can't get no justice! No respect!" These words of a protestor in Ferguson, Missouri, in August 2014 reflect a popular understanding of the close relationship between justice and respect.[7] This alliance of justice and respect for persons is evident in the scholarly realm as well. Nearly a half century ago, the philosopher Edward Kent argued that the "primordial meaning" of justice "is the specific claim for 'respect for person.'"[8] Subsequently, others have drawn various substantial relationships between these two ethical norms. In bioethics, this relationship has been advanced in regard to medical research, perhaps most substantially in recent reconsiderations of *The Belmont Report: Ethical Principles and Guidelines for the Protection of Human Subjects of Research.*[9] Produced in 1978 by the National Commission for the Protection of Human Subjects of Biomedical and Behavioral Research and in response to morally egregious medical research, *The Belmont Report* articulates three moral principles to guide ethical research: respect for persons, beneficence, and justice. In a 2005 collection of commentaries on *The Belmont Report*, titled (in short) *Belmont Revisited*, Larry Churchill argues that respect for persons is inaptly framed in the 1978 report as one moral principle among the three. "Justice," Churchill declares, "is not a weighty principle unless we assume that all subjects in research are equally entitled to our respect as fellow human beings. . . . No one is entitled to greater moral respect than others." Accordingly, he recommends that the principle of respect for persons be reframed as an "ontological claim," a "foundational commitment," and an "overarching value," rather than ranked equally with the other two principles.[10]

In a similar fashion, respect for persons undergirds my notion of community justice in health care. Beyond medical research, scant ethical attention has been brought to bear on this respect-justice connection in the health care realm. More specificity about respect for persons follows in my accounts of the moral criteria of community justice, but for present purposes, by "respect for persons" I mean the recognition that persons have inherent and equal moral worth, sometimes called "dignity." Respect for persons, offers Margaret Farley, is "the moral response appropriate to and required by this radical personal dignity or worth."[11] Based on recognition of the inherent value of persons, and found in numerous religious and philosophical worldviews, this respect for persons is commonly identified as "recognition respect" and is contrasted with "appraisal respect," in which respect is a response to the specific achievements of a person.[12]

In community justice the persons subject to this recognition respect are not the typical autonomous persons of bioethics, who are considered independent and due respect simply because of their capacity for autonomy. Informed by feminist thinkers across various disciplines, community justice recognizes persons as inherently situated, interdependent, and relational members of morally significant communities and groups. Such relationality renders a richer notion of respect for persons than the conventional respect for autonomy.[13] As Karen Lebacqz declares in her contribution to *Belmont Revisited*, "We are born into relationships and would not grow without them. We become who we are in community." She advises expanding the scope of respect for persons to "include respect for those communities and their traditions."[14] Notably, at least five other commentators in *Belmont Revisited* recommend a more relational interpretation of respect for persons;[15] or greater analytical attention to social groups, especially oppressed groups;[16] or the addition of a new *Belmont* principle, respect for communities.[17] "Ecological subjects," is how Lisa Eckenwiler describes such persons: "creatures whose identities and dwelling places are not merely relational but intersubjectively constructed, indeed, mutually constitutive."[18] As put by Larry Rasmussen, "We are essentially and not accidentally community moral beings."[19]

Robin Dillon's concept of "care respect" is especially fitting for this vision of community justice in health care as it "joins individuals together in a community of mutual concern and mutual aid, through an appreciation of individuality and interdependence."[20] As a variant of recognition respect, care respect acknowledges persons as having equal moral worth rooted both in their capacity for autonomy and in their particularities, including their similarities and differences in relation to others.[21] To say that all persons have equal moral worth speaks to a commonality, but this commonality does not make us generic persons deserving of generic respect. Rather, each person as a particularly situated person deserves particular respect, that is, respect shaped by our particularities. Similarly, self-respect demands that one attend to one's own particularities, to self-understanding, and to self-care.

Community justice rests on an obligation to respect persons that, as Farley puts it, "requires that we honor their freedom and respond to their needs, that we value difference as well as sameness, that we attend to the concrete realities of our own and others' lives."[22] The lyrics of Aretha Franklin's 1967 recording—"R-E-S-P-E-C-T, find out what it means to me"—affirm the importance of this contextual respect.[23] The song's deep resonance and enduring popularity suggests the magnitude of disrespect for particular persons in particular communities over time, as reiterated fifty years later in the words of the Ferguson protestor.[24]

The word "respect" has etymological roots in *respicere*, "to look again."[25] To respect is to attend closely or, as Dillon says, to respond with "perceptive attention": "The person who respects something pays attention to it and perceives it differently from someone who does not and responds in light of that perception." In turn, disrespect is signaled by "being oblivious or indifferent to it, ignoring or quickly dismissing it, neglecting or disregarding it, or carelessly or intentionally misidentifying it."[26] Many claims of injustice in health care point to disrespect, and specifically to the disrespect experienced by members of marginalized, nondominant groups, enacted by members of relatively powerful, dominant groups or the institutions and structures they have established. Examples include women whose reproductive health needs are not "seen" by lawmakers, women of color whose reproductive health needs are not taken seriously by white women and lawmakers, people with disabilities whose understandings of health and ability are dismissed by the able-bodied, and queer persons whose bodies and lives are pathologized by straight persons. At stake here, among other things, is the question of whose understandings or meanings of social goods, including health and health care, are recognized, valued, and ultimately respected.

A powerful link between justice and respect for persons is found in Michael Walzer's theory of complex equality, where justice is understood as respect for the particular meanings given to social goods:

> We are all (all of us) culture-producing creatures; we make and inhabit
> meaningful worlds. Since there is no way to rank and order these worlds
> with regard to their understanding of social goods, *we do justice to actual*
> *men and women by respecting their particular creations.* And they claim
> justice, and resist tyranny, by insisting on the meanings of social goods
> among themselves. Justice is rooted in the distinct understandings of
> places, honors, jobs, things of all sorts, that constitute a shared way of
> life. To override those understandings is (always) to act unjustly.[27]

For Walzer, the "meaningful world," the "shared way of life," and the creations that deserve respect and justice are those of the national political community.[28] That said, Walzer recognizes that "sometimes political and historical communities don't coincide, and there may well be a growing number of states in the world today [1983] where sensibilities and intuitions aren't readily shared; the sharing takes place in smaller units. And then, perhaps, we should look for some way to adjust distributive decisions to the requirements of those units."[29] "Perhaps" is the operative word here, for ultimately Walzer does not recognize subnational communities as creators of shared meanings that contribute to a shared way of life or as deserving of respect or justice.

Although Walzer remains committed to justice as respect for shared meanings as national creations, his justice-respect framework is relevant to thinking about community justice in health care and is exemplified in Emanuel's focus on community-based conceptions of the good life. Emanuel argues for respecting community-level meanings: "Justice is not realized by comparing entitlements to individual services, but by respecting the community's particular conception of the good life expressed in its distribution of goods."[30] But as I argued in the last chapter, Emanuel frames these good-life communities without respect for their internal diversity. As such, these communities function much like Walzer's nation in obscuring the particular creations of all community members. In contrast, community justice in health care insists on respect for the meanings and values that diverse communities create and hold dear.

A Possible Institutional Context

In support of a lucid description and understanding of the moral vision of community justice, I begin with a national vision, that is, a sketch of a national health care system that is potentially capable of enabling and reflecting community justice. As health care is a multilayered social good, just health care requires integrated institutional structures at the national, community, and other levels. Community justice is not attainable within the current organizational and financing arrangements of U.S. health care and thus requires institutional structures beyond the status quo. The institutional vision that follows is *not the necessary or even the desired* national health care system for community justice, but such a national vision helps to contextualize community justice.

Imagine the United States divided into geographically defined health care communities, roughly substate areas that may or may not mirror existing political or health care institution boundaries. Membership in the health care community would be based on one's presence or residency in a community, not on formal political membership based on citizenship or on economic status based on the ability to pay for health care. As such, health care communities are inclusive of all persons living within defined geographic parameters. Importantly, each health care community is made up of multiple and diverse communities: communities of color, religious and cultural communities, and so forth. The size of a health care community, as measured by geography or membership, would depend on the optimal conditions in a specific area for operational feasibility given the health care services to be offered and for effective community participation.[31] Rural health care communities would likely have relatively few members, whereas metropolitan areas would have many health care communities.

An elected community health board would be responsible for the negotiation of most community understandings of health and health care, the assessment and prioritization of the community's health care needs, and the provision of care to community residents. Some types of health care (elaborated below) would be provided at the national level. Community member participation in determining the nature and meanings of their community's health care is essential; this would be promoted intentionally through various means, including elected representation; direct participation in committees, councils, and coalitions; and health activism.

Communities would work with the national level of the health care system to determine community boundaries and the financing and delivery of care. They would participate in setting the national health budget, and community health boards would receive annual capitated payments from a national health care trust fund to finance the delivery of health care services in communities. The amount of payment would be based on the number of community members and overall community health status. The national trust would be financed collectively through a health care tax on persons, and a national budget for health care would be determined based on the aggregate needs of communities and health care's relative priority among other important social goods.

Each community resident would choose a particular health care provider responsible for providing them with a largely community-defined set of health care benefits. The community may define multiple packages of benefits compatible with agreed-to understandings of health and health care. Community health boards would pay providers an annual capitated fee to care for defined persons. These boards would also certify providers to practice in their communities and would collect data relevant to quality assurance. Multiple communities may work together to address common health problems and to consolidate certain functions such as provider certification and data collection.

Communities do not exist as discrete entities unto themselves—they are nested within multiple relations with other communities and the nation. A critical question arises regarding the roles of the different levels of collectivity in relation to justice: What are the health care concerns and responsibilities of the community? of the nation? My approach is one of shared responsibility and thus requires sorting the goods and services of health care roughly by degree of relationality and assigning them as the responsibilities of different collectivities. In this just health care system, communities would have responsibility for the creation and distribution of the more relational goods, for example, primary health care and public health activities, while the creation and provision of scarcer, less relational goods such as advanced surgery and other tertiary care would be a national responsibility.

Health care relationships, as relatively intimate, immediate, and ongoing, are best created at the community level: A primary-care visit with a local practitioner is likely to be more relational than a consultation with a specialist surgeon. The local practitioner will more likely know the patient's health history and current life situation and have a continuing commitment to a particular patient. A highly technically trained specialist may be located in a distant regional medical center and have a relatively brief interaction with the patient. This is not to say that such practitioners do not care or that they do not offer competent care; this care is less relational and less reliant on particular caring relationships than are some other health care goods. Also, tertiary care is relatively uncommon and more resource intensive compared to other types of health care and as such would be financially unfeasible for many health care communities. Furthermore, tertiary care centers serve relatively large populations and areas that are incompatible with meaningful participation in defining and distributing these services.[32]

The nature and limits of community-level decision making are identifiable in relation to three *national* standards of justice to which all just health care communities must abide: The first, just addressed, is that tertiary care services are defined and allocated at the national level. The second criterion entails the nationalized financing of this community-based health care system. A national budget for health care would be determined at the national level, and all persons would contribute to the national trust fund based roughly on their income. Monies would be allocated to communities on the basis of relative community need, as determined by the number of members and their health needs. This health care system, like that proposed by Emanuel, separates the financing of care from its provision: Communities define and provide care with resources collected and distributed nationally. This universal financing mechanism helps to assure that relatively unhealthy and/or low-income communities receive resources proportionate to their needs.

Community justice, the third national standard of justice, requires us to create health care governance structures that enable the effective voices of all persons in determining a community's understandings of health care. Community justice endeavors to change unjust community relations by requiring health care communities to abide by three moral norms or standards in their processes of creating mutually respected understandings of health and health care. These standards are inclusive, geographic health care communities; the provision of whole-person health care; and participation as effective voice in health care decision making. This moral vision of community justice does not assume that communities now hold shared or agreed-to understandings of health and health care. Nor does it aim for community understandings and values to be internally homogeneous and externally incommensurable, like those in Emanuel's good-life communities. Rather, the meanings and understandings of health care that community justice calls us to respect emerge from the engagement and deliberations of multiple communities within the health care community. Predictably this process of engagement will involve differences, conflicts, and overlapping understandings and commitments. Relatedly these community understandings will exist in close relationship to one another and to national understandings.

Given the inevitably varied understandings and values present in a health care community, how do communities create understandings and values that are genuinely "shared," in the sense of being agreed to? How might communities work together to create a just health care system? Community justice functions, in part, to identify and describe (at least some of) the institutional and policy conditions necessary for communities to determine their communal understandings and meanings of health care. Community justice does not describe in a fine-grained way what just health care would look like; rather, it articulates standards or norms required for reaching agreed-to understandings of health and health care that are needed for the provision of just health care services.

The Moral Vision: Three Ethical Norms

Three norms of community justice function as ethical criteria at the community level regarding the nature of community, of care, and of participation. These norms define the range of allowable community understandings and activities for just health care: (1) Each geographically defined community is inclusive of all persons within the community. (2) Health care is care for the whole person. And (3) participation in health care decision making requires the effective voices of multiple and diverse communities within the health care community. Community justice employs these three standards in an effort to organize health care such that it respects the equal moral worth of all persons in their particularities, including in their identities as community members. Community justice is both "universal" in its application of these three norms to all U.S. communities and "particular" in its effort to respect the distinct understandings of the various communities within the geographic health care community.

Just Community as Inclusive Geographic Communities

The core community of community justice consists of all residents in a defined geographic area. Residency, or where one lives, is characterized by a person's usual embodied presence in a particular place.[33] Financial resources and citizenship status are irrelevant to that community membership. Each resident is a member of a health care community. "All in" is another way of expressing the radical inclusivity of community justice—an inclusivity required by the fundamental obligation to respect the equal moral worth and dignity of all persons.

Critically, each geographic health care community is a community of multiple and diverse communities that work together to agree on the nature and scope of health care to be offered. I use the terms "geographic community" and "health care community" to represent this overarching community of communities. All geographic community members are morally relevant to just health care and are encouraged to participate in the communal process of meaning making.

A geographic community, rather than other sorts of communities, is the paradigmatic form of community in community justice because it facilitates inclusivity in four ways. First, the membership of geographic communities is more clearly definable than that of most other communities. This is particularly important when what is at stake is the creation and distribution of as valuable a social good as health care. Other types of communities have even more porous and fluid membership boundaries. Cultural, racial, ethnic, and religious communities, for example, are bound by persons' features and experiences, with fluctuating degrees of identification and commitment, thus rendering the scope of membership somewhat ambiguous for the just provision of a needed good. Membership in other communities such as the workplace and the professions is also liable to shift relatively frequently, given changing employment options and personal interests and goals. Furthermore, most persons are members of multiple identity and interest communities but typically only one geographic community. Despite population mobility, at a given moment, geographic communities have relatively plainly defined boundaries compared to other sorts of communities. This clarity of geographic boundaries led the Institute of Medicine nearly two decades ago to affirm geographic communities as a feasible and appropriate social grouping for monitoring health problems and measuring interventions, noting that, "although geographic (or civic) boundaries cannot adequately capture all of the potentially meaningful communities to which individuals might belong, they are a practical basis for analysis within the limits of current data systems."[34]

Second, most geographic communities are at least somewhat heterogeneous in that they are composed of multiple communities that historically have played strong roles in meaning making regarding health and health care, for example, religious, cultural, and medical professional communities.[35] Communal negotiation and deliberation involving the multiple and diverse understandings of these communities—each with its own internal heterogeneity—is a necessary condition for the creation of mutually agreed to understandings of health and health care.

Third, as described in chapter 1, health is strongly associated with the conditions of place, that is, with the physical, economic, and social environs within defined geographies. Jim Ife makes the case that "from an ecological perspective it can be argued that community should always be locationally based, because of the importance of the whole ecosystem, and the need for human communities to be integrated with the physical environment and the land."[36] To the extent that health status is influenced by the conditions of place, which includes the interdependent social fabric of multiple communities, it is coherent to engage persons in those places in determining the meanings and values of health and health care to them.

Finally, the provision of U.S. health care has been more closely associated with local geographic communities than with other sorts of communities.[37] It is no surprise that most persons seek their health care close to home. Community hospitals and community health centers are classic examples of health care institutions created by, and to serve, local geographic communities. While some religious communities—for example, the Catholic Church—have been significantly involved in the provision of care, they do not restrict care to their religious community members; they offer care to local community members, giving even these nongeographic communities a significant geographic dimension. That said, not all geographic communities have been inclusive of all residents. As noted in chapter 1, it was precisely the exclusionary practices of early local hospitals—often based on race, ethnicity, or religion—that prompted the establishment of hospitals by marginalized, often immigrant, communities committed to respecting the linguistic, cultural, and religious practices of their community members.[38]

These four reasons combine to justify geographic communities as the most inclusive and, accordingly, the most potentially just communities for health care. In community justice, all persons residing in a defined geographic community would be eligible not only to receive health care services but also to participate in creating the understandings of health and health care on which those services are based and, thus, to define "just health care" in their community. This geographic health care community does not begin with an assumed set of shared understandings, nor does it begin as just. The many different communities in the United States may well share some understandings given their common location within the wider society, but what these might be is known only through dialogue between them. The geographic community posited in my view of community justice for health care embraces differences and their contributions and challenges through the recognition and inclusion of multiple constituent communities.

One challenge to community justice's vision of inclusive geographic health care communities is the regular inattention, or even resistance, to the heterogeneity of communities. Feminist scholars and others have critiqued notions of community that homogenize, exclude, and thus obscure the actual "we" of communities.[39] Elizabeth Frazer and Nicola Lacey's articulation of the problem warrants lengthy quotation:

> Both common sense experience and sociological interpretation tell us that modern societies are made up of multiple "communities-within-communities" . . . all of which generate meanings, evaluations, norms, expectations and so on. This cultural heterogeneity has been underemphasised by communitarians because of its inconsistency with the cosy, pre-modern conception of community from which the *ideal* of community gets much of its rhetorical force, and because of fears about a multiplicity of mean-generating communities leading to fragmentation and incoherence in the communitarian picture of the world. Of course, this kind of fragmentation is indeed a threat to social order if it is thought to entail that there is simply no way of making sense of ourselves, of reconciling our differences, of living peaceably together. But, at a sociological level, this kind of fragmentation is precisely what we are confronted with in the modern (or perhaps post-modern) world, and the great political challenge we face is to learn to manage it in ways which do not deny our interdependence, repress difference or seek stability via the institutionalisation of unjust inequality in ways which construct such inequality as "normal" or "natural." [40]

A clear example of community membership restriction in the United States is the exclusion of undocumented residents from most publicly funded health care programs.[41] The eleven million undocumented immigrants living in the United States make up the largest group of residents ineligible for federal health care programs, including the Patient Protection and Affordable Care Act insurance plan subsidies plus tax credits and reductions in cost sharing, Medicaid (with the limited exception of emergency Medicaid), and the Child Health Insurance Program.[42] Reflecting the multilayered social nature of health care, this federal denial of these immigrants as members of the national health care "community" is being met with the recognition by a number of states, counties, and municipalities that undocumented immigrants are members by their state and local health care communities. For example, in June 2015, California governor Jerry Brown signed a budget bill that expanded Medi-Cal (California Medicaid) coverage to all income-eligible children regardless of immigration status.[43]

In a move that more directly challenges the federal exclusion, a group of California state lawmakers recently worked to gain state approval to seek a federal waiver that would allow California to open its state insurance exchange to undocumented immigrants, enabling them to buy lower-cost insurance plans available to other similarly incomed residents. "We are trying to come up with sensible, progressive policies that help to integrate every Californian," says state senator Ricardo Lara, sponsor of the state bill, in a clear declaration of the common state membership of all residents regardless of immigration status.[44] In summer 2015, the Huntington Park (California) City Council appointed two undocumented residents to city commissions, including Francisco Medina to the Health and Education Commission.[45] The purpose of the Health and Education Commission is "to create awareness of health and education matters in the City; determine health and education needs in the Community; and attempt to implement plans for improved health and education in the City."[46] In this move, Medina was officially recognized—not as a recipient of public services, not as a member of the undocumented community, but as a member of the municipality with an important voice in defining that community's health needs and improving its health.

Community justice, by including all residents and their communities within a geographic community, supports the heterogeneity of the health care community necessary for the two other justice criteria: whole-person health care, and effective voice in community decision making.

Just Care as Whole-Person Care

In community justice, just health care must attend to whole persons, both sick and healthy. This two-part criterion—care for whole sick persons and care for whole well persons—puts broad parameters on the scope of health care that communities must offer. But within those bounds health care communities negotiate the more specific meanings and practices that they understand to be whole-person care.

"Caring," says Daniel Callahan, "is the foundation stone of respect for human dignity and worth upon which everything else should be built."[47] This ethical demand for whole-person care ultimately rests on the obligation to respect for persons in our wholeness, which is to say, in our commonalities and in our differences. Health care is an expression of human interdependence, a multitude of interpersonal and institutional responses to human need and vulnerability, and healing relationships that, at best, restore a person's wholeness and integrity. In *Compassionate Respect* Farley expresses that "to care for a person adequately and genuinely as a person is to care for her in relation—in the context of the story of her relationships, past, present, and future."[48] To care justly is to understand a person as the intersectional nexus of relations of gender, race, sexuality, class, and more and as a member of multiple communities that shape both that person's health and health care needs. To care for whole persons is to attend perceptively to the relations within which persons live, including the relations of power, privilege, and oppression. Echoing Dillon's notion of care respect, Barbara Herman asserts, "To be responsive to need requires that one knows what it looks like. . . . Once we go beyond urgent need, [understood as universal], the nature and status of different needs becomes increasingly local and context dependent."[49] Whole-person care, therefore, requires health care practitioners who can understand many particular needs and are able to competently respond to them.

Responding to the full complement of a sick person's needs is a challenge to the individualistic, disease-oriented, treatment-centered biomedical model as well as to the economic incentives and efficiency goals of the current U.S. health care system. In a powerful narrative about the limits of contemporary health care, family physician Colleen T. Fogarty describes her "Jiffy Boob" experience at a breast care center: "Although I am in the most 'women-centered' mammography place in town, I'm left with the feeling that I'd been through a 'breast mill,' passing among many staff members performing single tasks as they send me through their assembly line."[50] Fogarty's experience resonates with Eric Cassell's observation nearly four decades earlier that the first year of medical education is about the "disintegration" of the person/patient into complex biological systems and involves "[approaching] the body as an object—a body completely depersonalized, stripped of those awesome aspects that constitute the unique nature of individuals."[51] Among health care practitioners a growing "whole-person care" movement is attempting to counter this reductionist focus,[52] but as one medical school dean recently lamented, contemporary medicine remains "radically incomplete, despite staggering scientific progress."[53]

This radical incompleteness of medicine can be harmful. In an eloquent narrative of the health care system's failures in the life of Eva, a relatively healthy eighty-seven-year-old woman, geriatrician Louise Aronson is clear: "Those who argue that health care consists primarily of prescriptions and procedures, or treatment of body parts and diseases, have created a system that prioritizes medicine to the detriment of patient health." [54] Aronson's group practice offered Eva an alternative—a more whole-person model of care, in which "the geriatrician would manage her diseases as her previous doctors had, but he or she also would begin by establishing Eva's life and health priorities, address her function and transportation challenges, review her medications and appointments to see if all were truly necessary, and be available by phone or to make a home visit if she got sick to try and prevent hospitalizations." [55] Such a model of clinical care better approaches the whole-person care required of community justice as well as affirms the care respect that ethically undergirds it.

As noted, to care for sick persons as whole persons is to respond to them in *"person terms,"* not in *"body terms."*[56] Just care requires that caregivers and institutions be capable of attending to sick persons as multidimensional beings with deeply intertwined physical, psychological, cultural, social, and spiritual/religious needs.[57] It involves health care practitioners who understand how a sick person is relationally connected to the world and how that sick person envisions what it means to be whole and healthy, to be cared for, and by whom. At the least, just health care means broadening the scope of disease-centric biomedicine that envisions each patient as a "presenting problem." Nursing philosophies of care typically assume a more complex patient than does the biomedical model, and similar to social workers, chaplains, mental and behavioral health counselors, nurses are trained to offer relatively holistic care.

Rarely can a single, even holistic, care giver meet all the needs of a sick person. Multidisciplinary teams of culturally competent and congruent care givers, professional and nonprofessional, from biomedical and other cultural healing systems, must work together to meet the range of patient needs. A growing cadre of care givers, community health workers, translators, and health care advocates are attending to previously neglected needs such as culturally competent care, transportation, and support in negotiation of the health care system. One implication of just whole-person care is that its responsibilities are somewhat open-ended. As a sick person's life situation and needs change, so, too, does the nature of a just response. Thus, just health care requires particularly flexible teams and caregivers.

Another implication of whole-person care is that the hierarchical ordering of care givers that gives physicians "occupational dominance"—and thus impedes whole-person care—would need to change.[58] Empirical research by Lucian Leape and colleagues reveals in graphic detail how the disrespectful behaviors of physicians not only humiliate and demean nurses, medical students, residents, and patients, they also risk patient safety, in part through inhibiting competent teamwork among the clinical staff.[59]

Finally, health care in the United States continues to privilege biomedicine and its norms, practitioners, and institutions despite the fact that many persons hold health beliefs and engage in healing practices of more than one healing system.[60] They may see a nurse practitioner and a cultural healer, a physician and a yoga therapist, or they may pray and take herbal remedies in addition to prescription medicines. Assuming that not all communities have the biomedical model at the center of their understandings of health and wholeness, just health care calls for a more diverse and integrated range of healing practitioners and institutions. Just health care in some communities will mean, for example, collaborating with indigenous traditional medicine healers, respecting religious healing practices, and the integration of diverse healing systems.

The second key component of whole-person care is whole healthy person care—that is, care that proactively attempts to keep persons well and, in that effort, promotes the social conditions for health. Integrated with local public health efforts, a holistic health care system would not only expand preventive care and health maintenance efforts within the practitioner-patient encounter, it would also actively promote health outside of it through, for example, needs assessments to identity the particular needs of all residents. Wellness-oriented care might also mean establishing mechanisms for identifying and monitoring key elements of residents' health status, as is done, for example, in many communities regarding childhood immunizations. Public health efforts to assure that children receive appropriate immunizations at the appropriate times are reinforced by state laws requiring that children entering school meet a certain immunization standard. This type of effort could be expanded to address multiple aspects of health, with or without the force of law.

Care for healthy persons entails care for healthy communities, indicating that just care must address the social/community determinants of health, including the social inequities that contribute to unhealthy lives. Significant institutional changes to the current health care system would be required, as would a significant shift in the understanding of health, from health as created primarily by individual factors to health as fundamentally shaped by social structural and institutional conditions. Accordingly, changes in health professions education would be needed to establish this broader understanding of health—for example, through education for structural competency, that is, medical competency in the social determinants of health.[61]

Just Participation as Effective Voice

The third standard of justice to which all health care communities must adhere is just participation understood as effective voice.[62] Community justice requires the just participation of community members in creating the social meanings, institutions, and conditions necessary for just (whole-person) health care. Just participation means that democratic deliberative conditions are in place that enable all community members to advocate for their particular understandings of health and health care and that the health care community seriously considers these understandings as it decides what health care it will establish and maintain for its community members.

Interestingly, the notion of justice as participation finds long-standing articulation and support in both Catholic moral theology and in feminist political philosophy. In Catholic moral theology, participation is both a necessary good and an obligation; social justice is "participation in the common good," says Lisa Sowle Cahill.[63] David Hollenbach elaborates this point in his work on human rights:

> Social justice is the measure which orders personal activities in a way which is suitable for the *production and protection* of the common good. . . . The aggregative concerns which fall under social justice do not begin with the presupposition that public good already exists or will come to exist spontaneously. . . . [Social justice] calls for the creation of those social, economic conditions which are necessary to assure that the minimum human needs of all will be met and which will make possible social and political participation for all.[64]

This Catholic understanding of social justice typically focuses on the role of government in shaping institutions toward the achievement of a national common good, though, as J. Bryan Hehir has noted, "The obligation to pursue [social justice] falls, in different ways, upon all in society: the state, voluntary associations, business and professional groups, religious and cultural organizations, and citizens themselves."[65] This Catholic conception of social justice as participation is a useful reminder of the multilayered institutional and political dimensions of just health care. Community justice does not start with a particular notion of the community common good because developing community-created understandings of health and health care is precisely the work of community justice.

Feminist political philosophers, too, have understood social justice as the institutional enablement of participation for all persons: "In the absence of a philosopher-king with access to transcendent normative verities, the only ground for a claim that a policy or decision is just is that it has been arrived at by a public which has truly promoted the free expression of all needs and points of view."[66] Every person should have the means to participate effectively in the health care decisions of their community. Similarly, Nancy Fraser argues for a concept of justice as "parity of participation," where justice is both a substantive principle and a procedural standard. As a substantive principle, justice allows that social arrangements are just "only if they permit all the relevant social actors to participate as peers in social life"; as a procedural standard, justice requires "the assent of all concerned in fair and open processes of deliberation, in which all can participate as peers."[67]

These overlapping Catholic and philosophical perspectives also similarly understand unjust participation as marginalization. "Marginalization, or lack of participation," Hollenbach notes, "becomes a primary criterion for judging if human dignity is being violated. Lack of adequate nourishment, housing, education and political self-determination are seen as a consequence of this lack of participation."[68] Citing marginalization as "perhaps the most dangerous form of oppression," Iris Marion Young asserts that "most of our society's productive and recognized activities take place in contexts of organized social cooperation, and social structures and processes that close persons out of participation in such social cooperation are unjust."[69]

Health care as a deeply relational and universally important good requires the interdependent participation of community members. Resonating with these Catholic and feminist perspectives, community justice obliges community members to participate in creating the conditions and institutions necessary for the just caring of all community members. More specifically, this just participation is understood to mean effective voice. To have effective voice signifies that community members mutually express their perspectives, seriously consider and attempt to understand the views of others, and reconsider and possibly revise their own views. A more definitive positive standard of just participation as effective voice is difficult to discern, as its meaning is partially community specific. Nonetheless, I can say more about the elements of effective voice in general terms.

Typically, the institutional means to effective voice will involve some community-tailored version of strong or participatory democracy.[70] Yet Frazer and Lacey warn that "our experiences as women should remind us . . . of the dangerously utopian conclusions about the virtues of participatory democratic structures that sometimes flow from discourse ethics. Formal rights of participation can all too easily serve to disguise inequalities of substantive access to speech and to being heard."[71] Supporting this point, a recent study by Christopher Karpowitz and colleagues found that gender inequalities in deliberative participation could be reduced by redesigning the deliberation procedures.[72] Community justice would require establishing mechanisms of democratic decision making that reduce inequities in participation.

An obvious prerequisite for effective voice is that members must "show up" in the health care community: They must participate in the conversation—oral, written, or other—and bring their commonalities and particularities to this community justice work.[73] As noted, just participation as effective voice must recognize and address power differentials within and among communities that enable some persons to express their views and values more freely and fully than others. "In the non-ideal community of discourse, which is the political world, who has the power, not only to speak, but to be heard?" ask Frazer and Lacey.[74] Or, in the words of John Stone, "What would it mean for one's voice to have a fair hearing"?[75] Notably, discussions of procedural justice in deliberative democracy in the health care realm often grant significantly more attention to speech than to listening: more attention to who is speaking and the reasonableness or legitimacy of their arguments than to who is paying attention and the quality or seriousness of that attention and subsequent consideration.

In a country rife with complex social relations undermined by privilege and oppression along racial, ethnic, gender, class, and other lines, it is no surprise that many communities know little and understand even less about one another. Recall that the principle of respect undergirding community justice requires perceptive attention, including, to paraphrase Robin Dillon, "trying to see persons clearly, as they really are in their own right, and not seeing them solely through the filter of one's own desires and fears or likes and dislikes."[76]

Effective voice requires that historically powerful groups—for example, organized medicine and health care policy elites—play a somewhat different role in decision making than marginalized groups historically excluded from participation—for example, communities of color, low-income persons, and uninsured persons. Various means of enhancing marginalized voices would have to be instituted through innovative institutional mechanisms to amplify the effective voices of these communities (more on this follows). Just participation as effective voice means that all communities must express their perspectives. But dominant groups in particular would need to be aware of their subordinating tendencies and thus "check their privilege" by, at times, being silent. In her essay, "Respect: On Witness and Justice," Sara Lawrence-Lightfoot describes how a certain silence conveys respect: "I do not mean an empty distracted silence. I mean a fully engaged silence that permits us to think, feel, breathe, and take notice . . . a silence that gives the other person permission to let us know what he or she needs."[77] In Young's terms, "A respectful stance of wonder toward other people is one of openness across, awaiting new insight about their needs, interests, perceptions, or values."[78] The respect for persons that undergirds community justice requires such respectful silence and openness in recognition of the differentials in power, privilege, and respect now accorded various communities.

Beyond speaking and listening, effective voice requires a serious engagement with another's views, but not by trying to put oneself in another's shoes—which is not only impossible but also violates the obligation to respect persons in their particularities.[79] Nor can one understand others by making assumptions about them or by simply agreeing with them. "Questions," says Young, "can express a distinctive form of respect for the other, that of showing an interest in their expression and acknowledging that the questioner does not know what the issue looks like for them."[80] To respect, to look again, to seriously consider another's understandings, requires the hard work of deep listening, questioning, dialogue, and deliberation.

Finally, effective voice requires that community members reexamine their own views in light of other community members' views with the potential for individual change and communal agreement of particular health care understandings. "Wonder," says Young, "also means being able to see one's own position, assumptions, perspective as strange, because it has been put in relation to others."[81] Furthermore, "Through [dialogue] we also construct an account of the web of social relations that surrounds us and within which we act."[82] Effective voice helps to build the just community relations necessary for health care decision making.

At the present time, few structured means exist by which community members can express, consider, deliberate, and decide their understandings of health and health care. The effective voice of all communities within the health care community is necessary for the deliberation of meanings of health and health care, negotiation of agreed-to understandings, and allocation of community resources for care. Without multiple and diverse voices, there is, at best, weak deliberation and, consequently, only partial and ineffectual agreed-to understandings of health and health care. It is because community justice is, in significant measure, contingent on agreed-to understandings of health and health care that the conditions for effective voice of multiple communities must be institutionalized.[83]

Community members might participate in various official and unofficial institutions and structures as a means to effective voice, for example, as elected health board representatives, as self-help patient groups, and as community organizers, advocates, and activists. The community health board, as an elected representative body, would be the primary means through which many community members participate. All community members would have the opportunity to elect representatives who would, in turn, play a major role in determining the agreed-to understandings of health and health care and in governing the system of care to be established. The board would need to be structured in such a way as to represent the perspectives of all communities, perhaps through designated seats for marginalized groups or, as Stone suggests, through proportional representation.[84] In particular, communities would need to determine the role of historically dominant medical and health care professionals vis-à-vis "consumers" on the board.

Multiple other formal participatory structures could be employed: advisory groups, boards, commissions, focus groups, and town hall meetings. Participatory councils, assemblies, or coalitions within and among communities in a health care community are additional means of encouraging the effective voices of marginalized communities. Surveys, polls, and individual interviews alone are not suitable, as they typically lack the dialogic engagement necessary for effective voice.

Among patients, the chronically ill are often the most intimately involved patients in the health care system. Their relationships with individual providers and institutions are ongoing and relatively well developed, although these relationships are not necessarily a means of effective voice. Chronically ill persons know well the limits of an acute care–oriented health care system like that of the United States and are frequently frustrated in their attempts to get the care they deem necessary.[85] One means to their greater effective voice has been through their creation and participation in self-care/self-help groups and health movements.[86] Such groups have empowered the chronically ill, both individually and collectively, to challenge provider and community understandings of their experiences and needs. Thus, the establishment of patient groups is one possible institutional mechanism for creating effective voice among some community residents.

Given the exclusionary history of democratic deliberation, effective voice is likely to require additional consumer advocacy efforts and grassroots activism in order for marginalized groups to clarify, strengthen, and communicate their perspectives.[87] While formal structures of deliberative democracy are critical, they are unlikely to be sufficient for community justice in the current inequitable U.S. social, political, and economic context.[88] Grassroots activism, community organizing, and consumer advocacy networks could be additional mechanisms to voice community understandings and might engage petitions, protests, art, and music as vehicles for effective voice.

Collectively, community health boards and other formal mechanisms, patient groups, and consumer advocacy and activist groups offer diverse structures conducive to just participation as effective voice. Whether, in fact, these institutions would encourage just participation would reside in the many decisions yet to be made about their particular shape and implementation in a specific community.

Conclusion

Together, an inclusive geographic community, whole-person care, and effective voice set the standards of justice governing each community's health care activities. The institutions I propose here are an attempt to articulate some of the structural requirements of community justice and to contribute normatively and concretely to our understandings of justice in health care. In its respect for the particular understandings of health and health care created by multiple, diverse communities within a health care community, community justice is distinct from both Emanuel's liberal-communitarian proposal and the liberal theories of health care justice examined earlier. In community justice, just health care communities are well-defined, inclusive, and diverse geographic communities capable of the serious and sustained conversation and deliberation necessary for the discernment of agreed-to understandings required for just health care. These communities affirm the multiplicity of perspectives within them and engage them despite inevitable conflict. Furthermore, some communities share some common understandings and values and, for this reason, are capable of cooperation among themselves and with other institutions.

Community justice identifies the need for, and suggests concrete democratic conditions and institutions for, just participation as effective voice. Emanuel and others rely on current institutions and structures for democratic deliberation, neglecting, for example, biomedical and other forms of social dominance as serious obstacles to participation. Similar to Emanuel's vision, community justice recognizes that both the nation and geographic health care communities have discrete responsibilities in the definition and provision of health and health care.

The challenges of taking seriously our relationality, our obligations, and our communities in our thinking about health care justice are significant. With this moral and institutional vision of community justice in mind, I now turn to contemporary health care policies, programs, and other endeavors that, intentionally or not, express one or more of the three norms of community justice: an inclusive geographic community, whole-person care, and effective voice.

Chapter 5

Community Justice in U.S. Health Policy

Public policy is about communities trying to achieve something as communities. This is true even though there is almost always conflict within a community over who its members are and what its goals should be, and even though every communal goal ultimately must be achieved through the behavior of individuals.

—Deborah Stone

Communities have had long and significant roles in U.S. health policy. In the tellingly titled article "Paradigms Lost: The Persisting Search for Community in U.S. Health Policy," Mark Schlesinger tracks the shifting roles of geographic communities in health care and health policy since the mid-1600s.[1] Over time, communities have been responsible for the sick care of local residents; have controlled hospitals, dispensaries, health centers and established health planning processes; have been the objects of federal and state policies; and have had myriad lesser forms of engagement and participation in policies that shape the organization and financing of U.S. health care.

Communities continue to play influential if not well-recognized roles in early twenty-first-century health care. Despite the primary orientation of the Patient Protection and Affordable Care Act of 2010 (ACA) to the insurance status of individuals, the reform also has engaged communities in widely disparate ways. On the one hand, the ACA added $11 billion-plus for new and renovated health centers to serve residents of medically underserved areas, mandated that nonprofit hospitals complete triannual community health needs assessments of their local communities, and promoted a diverse group of delivery and payment reform efforts that seek to integrate local communities into successful health care reform.[2] On the other hand, Community Transformation health promotion grants to local communities were funded and then defunded, and members of certain religious groups—specifically health-care-sharing ministries—were wholly exempted from the individual mandate to carry health insurance.[3] In the context of contemporary health policy, the community justice framework outlined in the previous chapter evokes two questions: First, in what ways do current communities significantly interact with health care and health policy? And second, how do these community-relevant policies, programs, and inter- actions enable or inhibit community justice?

To answer these questions at least in part, I examine three significant community involvements: (1) federally funded community health centers, (2) community health needs assessments by nonprofit hospitals, and (3) community-based health advocacy groups. Brief historical overviews prime my assessments of these community involvements. As each effort holds unique promise for community justice, so, too, each is uniquely constrained in relation to it.

Community Health Centers

On their face, community health centers (CHCs) appear to be the quintessential institutional embodiment of community justice. Serving all residents in geo- graphically defined medically underserved areas, these federally funded, non- profit health centers are governed by patient-majority boards, provide a broad range of health care services, and offer substantial community benefits in eco- nomic, employment, and leadership terms. A closer examination of CHCs in historical and contemporary contexts and in light of community justice norms reveals a more complex portrait.

In 1965, as part of President Lyndon B. Johnson's "War on Poverty," the federal Office of Economic Opportunity (OEO) funded the first two neighbor- hood health centers (NHCs), as they were originally called. The OEO channeled federal grant monies through local Community Action Programs to medical schools, local hospitals, and health departments, which administered these early programs.[4] Tufts University Medical School was the first grant recipi- ent, and two faculty members, Drs. Count Gibson and H. Jack Geiger, initi- ated health centers in Boston's Columbia Point housing project and in rural Mound Bayou, Mississippi. The next year, OEO funded six more centers, and the numbers grew rapidly, to more than fifty in 1968 and one hundred in 1971.[5]

Neighborhood health centers were an innovative model of health care delivery that offered relatively comprehensive primary-care services to all area residents regardless of race, ethnicity, or income. These centers were designed to respond to the particular needs of their communities through community advisory and governing boards and to support community development through the employment and training of local community members. The federal Medicaid and Medicare programs were also established in 1965 and provided public financing for health care services needed by, respectively, eligible low-income persons (largely, mothers and children) and most adults aged sixty-five years and older. Some of these Medicaid and Medicare beneficiaries were NHC patients, and these reimbursements, along with federal health center grants and patient out-of-pocket payments, sustained the centers financially in their early years.

Health center supporters of the 1960s and 1970s held multiple and sometimes conflicting visions for these health centers. As Isabel Marcus observes, "advocates for the poor" understood health centers as a new form of health care delivery aimed at serving primarily low-income persons, while "sweeping reformers" held a more radical vision, one aimed at reforming the entire health care system as well as eliminating the social structures, including poverty and racism, that contribute to poor health status.[6] Geiger clearly articulated the latter, more radical vision. In addition to calling for health care to become more primary care oriented, more community based, and more community controlled, Geiger explained that "the initial neighborhood health center proposal articulated a still broader goal . . . ; social and political change to affect those powerful determinants of health status that lie in the economic and social order. Health care services, it was argued, should be deliberately used as a point of entry for such broader social change."[7] Alternatively, former OEO official Mildred A. Morehead expressed a more limited vision for these health centers: "The principal objectives as we saw them were to provide a new model of health care for the poor, to bring high quality of service in 'innovative' ways to the nation's disadvantaged. It is true that a number of objectives other than health care were encompassed. . . . But the reorganization of the entire health care delivery system was not in the minds of the persons I worked with."[8] This tension between broad social transformation and health care services to low-income and medically underserved persons surfaced in the first years of neighborhood health centers in, for example, debates and vacillating policy about the boundaries of "neighborhood"—was the neighborhood "all residents" or more narrowly "the poor"? That neighborhood health centers were to serve all residents was affirmed in 1972 federal legislation that also encouraged a more traditional medical model of care that eventually squelched the centers' potential for greater systemic and structural reform.

From 1965 to 1975, neighborhood health centers moved from a grand vision (that of serving twenty-five million people in one thousand centers by 1973), to near extinction (by means of budget cuts, patient means testing, and health care practice constraints), and finally to institutionalized survival ensured by federal legislation in 1975.[9] Policy makers' doubts about the efficacy and costs of the War on Poverty, including NHCs, were growing; some local medical providers resisted collaboration with NHCs, which they perceived as a threat to their patient base; and the radical implications of proposed social change through health care restructuring were becoming more obvious. In the early 1970s, the federal government transferred the NHC program from OEO to the Department of Health, Education, and Welfare (now the Department of Health and Human Services), and along with that shift came more obstacles to health center growth.[10] Not coincidentally, in 1971, health center supporters established the (now called) National Association of Community Health Centers (NACHC) to advocate on behalf of the health centers in Washington, DC.

President Richard Nixon's attempt to end federal support for health centers ultimately failed when Congress passed legislation in 1975 that specifically and permanently authorized, and then funded, community health centers. Commonly known as Section 330, this legislation, which in 2016 continues to authorize CHCs, also brought several other health programs under this health center umbrella, simultaneously consolidating and expanding health centers' reach and potential political support. The centers' new designation as "community" health centers distinguished neighborhood health centers, with their politically controversial pasts, from these seemingly novel, refreshed health centers. Alice Sardell observes that health centers endured this rocky period precisely because they were presented as "an effort to provide health services to a limited number of low-income people, rather than part of a larger program for general health system reform."[11] By the centers' ten-year anniversary, the vision of the advocates for the poor had largely prevailed over that of the sweeping reformers.

Forty years later, in 2015, after successfully enduring more difficult political and economic periods, health centers celebrated fifty years of operation.[12] Reflecting the health centers' considerable growth in number and in organizational and funding complexity, the terminology relating to these centers has also became more complicated.[13] "Health Center Program grantees," or "grantees," are nonprofit organizations or, in a limited number of cases, public agencies, that receive Section 330 funding for health centers to serve either all residents in a medically underserved community or all members of one of three particular underserved "special populations": migratory and seasonal farmworkers and their families, homeless persons, or public housing residents. The term "community health centers" technically refers to a subset of these grantees that serves all persons in a defined service area, though the term is sometimes used to signify all types of health centers. In 1989–1990, the Centers for Medicare and Medicaid Services (CMS) began certifying these grantees and other health centers to receive enhanced Medicare and Medicaid reimbursement, and centers with such certification were called "federally qualified health centers," or FQHCs.[14] "FQHC look-alikes" (FQHC-LAs) are also CMS certified, serve similar communities or populations, but do not receive Section 330 funding. Increasingly, the terms "health centers," "community health centers," and "FQHCs" are used interchangeably both inside and outside the health center sphere.[15]

In 2013, 1,202 Health Center Program grantees served 21.7 million patients in 9,170 delivery sites, roughly evenly split between urban and rural areas. Most patients (93 percent) had family incomes below 200 percent of the federal poverty level, 35 percent were uninsured, and 41 percent were Medicaid beneficiaries. These patients were disproportionately people of color: 24 percent were African American (whereas African Americans constitute just 14 percent of the U.S. population), and 35 percent were Latin@ (nationwide, Latin@s are 17 percent of the population).[16] In addition, one hundred FQHC-LAs (7.7 percent of all health centers) served over one million similar patients.[17] It is estimated that together these health centers will serve twenty-eight million persons in 2015.[18] Combined, health centers (grantees and non-grantees) constitute the largest group of primary-care providers in the United States, not to mention considerable strength in the health care safety net.[19]

Across their five decades, health centers have been remarkably resilient both politically and financially, owing in no small measure to NACHC and to their unusual support across the political spectrum.[20] As Robert W. Mickey put it in 2012, "It might be better to be lucky than good, but the health centers movement has been both, especially of late."[21] In 2008, President George W. Bush approved a large increase in health center funding, followed by the ACA's authorization of $11 billion in new health centers through 2015, later extended through 2017.[22] This ACA financial windfall led to the direct expansion of health center organizations, clinic sites, providers, services, and patients, while other ACA reforms, such as increased health insurance coverage of low-income persons through Medicaid and private plans, contributed indirectly to the health center expansion.[23] Today the health center program is, according to Mickey, "larger, financially more sure-footed, and more popular than ever before. It is also shouldering increasingly weighty expectations and public and political scrutiny."[24]

The multiple roles that communities play in health centers, plus the centers' sheer number and longevity, make the centers potentially influential promoters of community justice in three ways. First, to the extent that individual health centers provide health care services to all persons in designated service areas, they partially exemplify the geographic inclusivity required for community justice. Second, their comprehensive primary-care and enabling services enhance whole-person care, and finally, the patient-majority governing boards of health centers can serve as powerful vehicles for the voices of patients and community members.

Community justice requires that all persons in the United States are members of a health care community. As noted in the last chapter, one means of achieving this inclusivity would be to divide the entire U.S. population into geographically defined health care communities and have each health care community serve all residents within its bounds. Currently every community health center is open to serve all residents within a geographically defined service area that must also be designated as a medically underserved area. As such, health centers have a crucial, though limited, national coverage: In 2013, health centers served approximately 7 percent of the country's population (23 million of 319 million persons). While the inclusivity of each individual community health center aligns with community justice, the centers' partial coverage of the U.S. population only begins to approach it.

The collective reach of health centers is constrained by federal regulation regarding the types of communities eligible to receive health center funding. Each health center, by mission and legislation, must serve residents of a geographic area that has been federally designated as a "medically underserved area" (MUA) or serve members of a federally recognized medically underserved population group (MUP), specifically migrant and seasonal farmworkers, homeless persons, or public housing residents. Both MUA and MUP designations are established through an assessment of the area's medical service needs according to the Index of Medical Underservice (IMU). Four variables factor into an IMU score: the ratio of primary-care physicians to population, the infant mortality rate, the percentage of the population with incomes below the poverty level, and the percentage of the population aged sixty-five and older.[25] An IMU score of sixty-two or higher is required for a successful grant application.

The IMU was instituted in 1975, and despite many changes in U.S. health and health care over the last four decades, this methodology has remained unchanged. Given these four particular variables, it is not surprising that health centers are located in communities with large numbers of low-income Latin@s or African American residents. But one limitation of the IMU is that it identifies only certain types of medical need. For example, many persons with serious mental illness lack access to adequate health care services and, thus, can be reasonably considered to be medically underserved. Providers of mental health care have argued that this health care need is analogous to the needs of other populations groups, such as homeless persons, and therefore that persons with serious mental illnesses should likewise be designated a "special medically underserved population"[26] Notably, however, the four IMU variables do not identify mental health need. In another example, the Fenway Institute (Boston) has made the case that the significant unmet medical needs of the lesbian, gay, bisexual, and transgender (LGBT) population should qualify this group as "medically underserved." Yet the IMU formula as currently construed does not recognize the paucity of physicians knowledgeable about LGBT-specific health risks and needs, the stigma accorded and discrimination against these patients, and the dispersed nature of the LGBT population.[27]

A second IMU limitation is the inevitable "yo-yo effect" of this sort of means-tested program. Health centers must serve medically underserved areas and populations.[28] When they do so successfully, that is, when they reduce underservice—for example, by increasing the physician-population ratio—they become at risk of increasing their IMU score and losing the underservice designation required for federal funding, and thus they are at risk of closing. Absent the health center, the community is likely to once again become certifiably underserved and thus eligible to apply for health center funding.

In 2010, the ACA mandated a review of MUA/P and related designation methodologies, including the IMU. Earlier attempts to revise the methodologies in 1998 and in 2008 failed, in large measure owing to health center concerns that a revised formula would lead to a loss of MUA/P designation, and consequently a loss of funding, for some established programs.[29] The 2011 "Final Report" of the review recommends that the IMU be replaced with an Index of Primary Care Need that revises the four IMU index variables and grants each variable an assigned standard weight.[30] Rather than an absolute score threshold (e.g., sixty-two), one-third of areas or populations with the greatest need (as identified by the new index) would be designated "medically underserved" and thus eligible to receive federal health center funding.[31] Notably, while this revised index would better identify some primary-care needs, it still would not recognize persons with serious mental illness or the LGBT population as medically underserved.[32]

Since their start a half century ago, health centers typically have provided a comprehensive set of primary health services that extend well beyond the scope of care offered by most primary-care providers, that is, an expansive range of care that could serve to support whole-person care—this being the second aspect of community justice. At a minimum, health center grantees are required to offer basic primary-care services; diagnostic lab and radiology services; preventive medical and dental care, including perinatal services, family planning, well-child services, and many screenings; and referrals to medical specialty care and mental health and substance abuse services. Also required are enabling services that facilitate access to those primary-care services, including outreach, transportation, and translation services; case management, including program and financial eligibility assessment; and community education about the availability and use of health services.[33] As needed, health centers may provide behavioral, mental health, and substance abuse services (not simply referrals to them), recuperative care, and a wide array of environmental health services that reduce "unhealthful conditions." For example, responding to the occupational health needs of farmworkers, grantees offer work-related disease screening and injury prevention services.[34]

Numerous studies have shown health center care to be cost-effective and of high quality.[35] Typically, centers provide this care with a patient-centered team approach that may include community health workers, promotoras, and translators. Furthermore, they support care through referral relationships with area health care providers, including one or more hospitals. The most persistent gap in this range of care is the health centers' often insufficient and unreliable access to specialty care services. Even if health centers locate specialty services, they have scarce funds to pay for them. The ACA incentivizes health care providers to try new service-delivery models, for example, the Patient Centered Medical Home (PCMH) and the accountable care organization (ACO), with the goal of expanding patient access to more coordinated care across the spectrum of needed care. Health centers are increasingly adopting PCMH and ACO models in the quest for more integrated specialty care and more whole-person care, as well as for a reduction in health care disparities.[36] These innovations potentially mean greater collaboration with conventional health care providers through new, shared health information technologies such as electronic health records. Typically, conventional providers orient their care toward their patient populations rather than toward the wider community, and, as such, these new collaborations present tensions for health centers.

Whole-person care requires understanding and caring for a person's social, cultural, and relational needs for healing—as well as for their biomedical ones. Health centers are known for their linguistic and cultural responsiveness to the needs of the particular communities and populations they serve, and more is needed. In 2013, Latin@s constituted 35 percent of health center patients nationwide. A 2010 survey of over five hundred health center providers and staff serving Latin@ patients with diabetes across ten midwestern states found that the providers had "limited Spanish language ability and awareness of Latino cultural beliefs"—this, in an area that experienced nearly 50 percent growth in the Latin@ population in the decade ending 2010.[37] This same study found that providers understood little about different cultural subgroups among Latin@s or about the traditional treatments patients were using in addition to biomedical care.[38] Recent studies in New Mexico and Texas also identify significant Latin@ use of traditional medicine and complementary and alternative medicine, and many Latin@s do not inform their physicians of such use, suggesting room for more integrated whole-person care.[39]

The whole-person care of community justice requires attention not only to sick care but also to whole-person "health" care. To the extent that health centers provide preventive care services, such as immunizations, and address structural conditions in the community that impede health, they contribute to whole-person care. A recent NACHC initiative, Protocol for Responding to and Assessing Patient Assets, Risks, and Experiences (PRAPARE), is piloting an expanded patient social history to identify patients' experiences of the social determinants of health.[40] Such patient-centered efforts could be paired with parallel systemic-level data about community conditions: the economic, educational, political, housing, and food security conditions that affect much or all of the community. In another strategy that serves the whole person and echoes the early broad vision of neighborhood health centers, some health centers are mediating poor community health conditions and social inequities by working with social services agencies to help facilitate job training, housing assistance, and youth development.[41]

Perhaps the most distinctive feature of health centers is their governance by patient-majority boards, a form of consumer control that relates to the third norm of community justice: participation as effective voice.[42] Health center employees who are community members also have voice, but patient-majority governing boards offer the potential for unusually strong and effective community voice. Mandated by health centers' authorizing legislation, each center must have a governing board that is "composed of individuals, a majority of whom are being served by the center and who, as a group, represent the individuals being served by the center."[43] In practical terms, this means that 51 percent or more of board members must be currently registered health center patients who have had a health center visit within the last two years. Recent federal guidance on health center governance further clarifies that, "as a group, patient members of the board must reasonably represent the individuals who are served by the health center in term of race, ethnicity, and sex. Health centers are also encouraged to consider patient members' representation in terms of other factors such as socioeconomic status, age, and other relevant demographic factors."[44] A 2004 National Rural Health Association survey showed that 83 percent of board chairs were either patients or community members.[45]

The requirement for patient-majority boards assumes that communities have unique needs and resources that these boards will identify and that these boards will determine community-appropriate strategies for meeting those needs. Exemplifying community governance, health center boards are responsible for choosing the health center's executive director, approving the budget, determining the center's services and hours, and setting general organizational policies. It is notable that during the first decade of neighborhood health centers it was only after considerable struggle over the meanings of "community participation" that Congress wrote patient-majority governing boards into the federal legislation. The early OEO grantees—medical schools, hospitals, and public health departments—typically set up community advisory boards for input, but the 1975 health center legislation, responding to the demands of community members, shifted full control of health centers to community-based, patient-dominated governing boards.

A critical question is whether a patient-majority governing board necessarily leads to patient-dominant decision making and effective voice. Evaluations of governing boards are scarce, though recent research suggests that executive directors and physicians of centers have disproportionate power in defining and responding to community needs relative to board members[46] and that patient board members are of higher socioeconomic status than the "typical" patient population,[47] suggesting less than ideal patient representation and authority. Further study of board composition and actual operation is needed.

Most health center grantees are private nonprofit organizations, though up to 5 percent of health center appropriations may be granted to public agencies such as health departments, cities or counties, and universities. Known as "public centers," these health centers are subject to the same governance requirements as private health centers, but they are also bound by often-conflicting public governance laws. In these cases, a public center is required to establish a patient-majority "co-applicant" governing board, nearly identical to a nonprofit health center board, and together this co-applicant board and the public agency legally form the health center. This complicated mechanism is an attempt to maintain community control of health centers with public agency grantees, but the consequences of this arrangement are only beginning to be discerned.[48] In the current ACA context, as health centers increasingly affiliate with more conventional health care institutions both private and public and nonprofit and for-profit, concern is warranted about the future of community participation, not to mention legislated and effective community governance.

Health centers hold significant promise for advancing community justice. They promote an inclusive health care community by serving all residents in a geographic, medically underserved area; they offer wide-ranging services, including community-responsive enabling services; and they embody community governance via patient-majority boards. That said, health centers are limited to serving only MUAs and MUPs, a designation which currently excludes some underserved communities and groups, and, in various ways, ACA reforms threaten community governance. As health centers are encouraged by health system reforms to move toward becoming even more mainstream health care institutions, they risk losing their community roots—and potentially their positive role in community justice.

Community Health Needs Assessment and Community Benefits

Effective as of 2012, nonprofit hospitals in the United States have additional tax-reporting responsibilities by virtue of the ACA community benefit reforms embedded in Internal Revenue Service (IRS) tax policy. At least once every three years, each nonprofit hospital must undertake a community health needs assessment (CHNA) in order to substantiate its contributions or benefits to the local community and, thus, to justify its federal tax-exempt status. (State and local tax exemption policies have additional requirements.)

This federal obligation is the latest step in a long regulatory relationship between community hospitals and their federal tax status.[49] In the late nineteenth century, federal income-tax policy exempted nonprofit corporations with a charitable purpose for two reasons: Nonprofits paid the costs of activities that the government would otherwise be responsible for, and hospitals, in particular, offered a public benefit through the "promotion of the general welfare."[50]

Through the early twentieth century, nonprofit hospitals typically, if unevenly and inconsistently, fulfilled this purpose by providing some level of charity care—that is, by providing health care services without cost to patients unable to pay for them.[51] In 1956, the IRS set a federal standard requiring tax-exempt nonprofit hospitals "to provide as much charity care as they could afford."[52]

In 1969, given the ambiguity of the 1956 standard and the perception that the recently enacted Medicare and Medicaid programs would lead to fewer uninsured persons needing charity care, the IRS took a turn "toward community." It expanded the tax-exempt standard beyond charity care to individuals to also require "community benefits": services or activities that benefit the entire community, not only its indigent subset.[53] This new community benefits standard was accompanied by other procommunity requirements, including the establishment of a community-based board of directors and the provision of emergency-room services to all community members regardless of ability to pay.

Over the next several decades, the U.S. health care system transformed into an increasingly for-profit, competitive, market-driven industry. Health care institutions including hospitals merged, restructured, consolidated, and closed. Executive compensation soared, as did the number of uninsured persons—while charity care declined.[54] Congress observed the "ever-blurring lines between for-profit and not-for-profit hospitals" and in 2004 and 2006 held hearings on the tax-exempt status of nonprofit hospitals and their provision of charity care and emergency care, as well as their billing and collections practices in regard to uninsured persons.[55] In 2008, the IRS revamped Form 990, required of tax-exempt organizations, and added Schedule H for the reporting of hospital community-benefits activities and expenses. This standardized reporting has enabled research on community benefits that demonstrates, for example, that, in 2009, 85 percent of community-benefit expenditures of nonprofit community hospitals were for charity care services—and less than 0.5 percent for community-level health improvement activities.[56]

Codified in IRS tax policy, the ACA mandated several new community-benefits requirements applicable to the over 3,900 nonprofit and government community hospitals.[57] These requirements include institutional policies regarding financial assistance (formerly called "charity care"), accessibility of emergency medical care to all, and restrictions on disproportionate hospital charges, billing, and collection practices that disadvantage uninsured persons. In addition, the requirement for a community health needs assessment became effective under Proposed Guidelines in 2012. Final Rules for CHNAs were published in December 2014.[58] These nonprofit hospitals, which make up 80 percent of all

U.S. hospitals, must now report (via a newly revised Schedule H) two general categories of community benefit expenses: financial assistance to patients for health care services, and "other benefits," including "community health improvement services," community benefits operations, health professions education, and research. Here I focus on "community health improvement services," as the CHNA is the primary mechanism for establishing the need for these services.

The CHNA process requires that each hospital identify and prioritize "significant" community health needs and potential community resources for responding to those needs. In a required implementation plan (companion to the CHNA), the hospital must outline its strategies for, and its role in, addressing each of these needs or state why it is not doing so. Hospital authorities must approve both the CHNA and the related implementation plan, and the final CHNA report must be readily and publically available. Unlike the CHNA report, the hospital does not have to post its implementation strategy on a website; however, it must be file that plan with its IRS Form 990 and have it available for review at the hospital.

As with community health centers, the significant number and reach of nonprofit hospitals mean that CHNAs hold rich potential for promoting community justice. And, as with community health centers, the operational details will determine whether CHNAs will be more of an asset or an obstacle to community justice.

According to IRS regulations, the hospital determines the definition of community used in the needs assessment, though the regulatory guidelines suggest that the community should align with the hospital's service area and should not "exclude medically underserved, low-income, or minority populations who live in the geographic areas from which the hospital facility draws its patients." Here, medically underserved populations are defined as "populations experiencing health disparities or at risk of not receiving adequate medical care as a result of being uninsured or underinsured or due to geographic, language, financial, or other barriers."[59] As such, it is reasonable to expect CHNAs to address relatively inclusive geographic communities, though, like CHCs, CHNAs will not have national coverage.

Community health needs assessments hold particular promise for advancing whole-person care, both sick and well care, given the IRS definition of health needs as "requisites for the improvement or maintenance of health status both in the community at large and in particular parts of the community (such as particular neighborhoods or populations experiencing health disparities)." Thus, health needs are not limited to access to health care services and may include efforts "to prevent illness, to ensure adequate nutrition, or to address social, behavioral, and environmental factors that influence health in the community."[60] This wide interpretation of health needs reflects a growing understanding that personal health care services make a critical but finite contribution to health, that social determinants also decisively shape health, and that individual health is inextricably tied to population and community health. To the extent that nonprofit hospitals identify, prioritize, and address these whole-person and whole-community health needs, they could significantly foster the conditions necessary for community justice.

Importantly for whole-person care, the IRS allows that "some community building activities *may* also meet the definition of community benefit" and describes these community building activities as including housing, economic or workforce development, community support, physical and environmental improvements, leadership development and community member training, coalition building, and community health improvement advocacy.[61] Yet IRS Schedule H is vague about whether these critical efforts to address the underlying causes of poor health actually count as legitimate community benefit expenditures.[62] In response, Sara Rosenbaum has called for a safe harbor provision to ensure that these expenses are approved and thus incentivize hospitals in their community-wide efforts.[63] To the extent that CHNAs help hospitals better identify and respond to the needs of their communities, they have the ability to strengthen the whole-person care of their community members.

It is the community input into CHNAs that would seem to hold the most potential for the just participation as effective voice norm of community justice. The IRS mandates that hospitals "must solicit and take into account" community input from "persons representing the broad interests of the community," defined as three sources: (1) a governmental public health department at the regional, state, local, or tribal level; (2) "members of medically underserved, low-income, and minority populations . . . or individuals or organizations serving the interests of such populations;" and (3) written comments received about the hospital's most recently published CHNA and implementation strategy (not those in progress).[64] A hospital may solicit and take into account input from additional community persons or organizations, but it is not required to do so.

Yet this CHNA process sets up many barriers to community participation, not to mention effective voice.[65] No community input is required regarding the hospital's definition of community or regarding which community representatives the hospital selects for input. Hospitals do not have to make a draft CHNA report publically available for comment, nor do they have to respond to or dialogue with community members and organizations that submit input. The regulations do not require community input into the hospital's implementation strategy for meeting community health needs. One public comment to the Proposed Rules argues for mandated community input on the current draft CHNA so that a community knows that an assessment is in progress and so that the assessment "would yield findings more indicative of community priorities and provide a better framework for collaboration." The IRS declined this recommendation "due to the complexity of the additional timeframes and procedures such a process would require" and asserted that feedback on the prior CHNA report and implementation strategy "will result in a meaningful exchange over time and that the longer timeframe will both give the public sufficient time to provide comments (including comments reflecting changing circumstances) and give hospital facilities sufficient time to take the comments into account when conducting their next CHNA."[66]

The CHNA report is required to describe how the hospital took community member and organizational input into account, but that requirement can be fulfilled simply by including a written section that "summarizes, in general terms, any input provided by such persons and how and over what time period such input was provided."[67] In other words, the hospital need not articulate how community input was taken into account and prioritized; it need only describe the received input and when and how it was received. The hospital's CHNA report must be "widely available"—that is, it can be posted on a website, with a print copy available for inspection at the hospital—but the hospital does not need to translate the report and to proactively publicize it.[68]

Perhaps reflecting a weak expectation that the hospital would actually address the significant community health needs that it identifies, the IRS Final Rules list five reasons the hospitals may not address these needs: "resource constraints, other facilities or organizations in the community addressing the need, a relative lack of expertise or competency to effectively address the need, the need being of relatively low priority, and/or a lack of identified effective interventions to address the need."[69] It is not clear whether hospitals are accountable for achieving their implementation strategies or are accountable simply for completing the CHNA and implementation plan.

These participation concerns, combined with the weak support for substantive community input in the CHNA, raise serious questions about the ability of the CHNA to promote effective voice. Indeed, a 2015 review of thirty-eight Georgia CHNAs found that only 18 percent of hospitals "explicitly and intentionally gathered input from members of vulnerable populations."[70] Requiring hospitals to identify the health needs of their communities is vital to both individual health care services and to community health. Whether the present CHNA is a sufficiently strong mechanism to do this and thus to promote community justice remains to be seen.

Community Health Advocacy Groups

Many communities, whether united by geography, identity, or interests, are active shapers of contemporary health policy and health care, not only through community institutions such community health centers and through federal policy mandates such as hospital needs assessments, but also through the diverse efforts of community health advocacy groups. As varied as the communities they are embedded in, these groups engage in community health advocacy by "taking a position on [a community health] issue, and initiating actions in a deliberate attempt to influence private and public policy choices."[71] Well-known examples of health advocacy groups include Health Care for All, the Boston Women's Health Book Collective, GMHC (Gay Men's Health Crisis), and Not Dead Yet, a disability rights organization. Such dynamic collectivities form, grow, shrink, reform, merge, hybridize, and dissolve—and thus are difficult to categorize neatly. Several recent typologies of these groups offer overlapping descriptive categories, including patient groups, health activist groups, consumer advocacy groups, grassroots organizations, health movements, health access movements, embodied health movements, and constituency-based health movements.[72] A local group may grow into a regional, state, or national movement, and conversely, a national movement may motivate local collective action. Groups have varying levels of inclusivity, power, and privilege, and they sometimes compete for resources. Frequently formed in response to community experiences of oppression and injustice, some groups choose names that reflect their demands to be heard, for example, Raise Women's Voices, Hear Us Now, and SisterSong.

The philosophical frameworks and strategic approaches that guide health advocacy groups vary widely and often have intersecting histories, motivations, and goals; for example, community action, community participation, community control, community organizing, community development, community building, community empowerment, community partnerships, community-oriented primary care, and community-based participatory research. Specific tactics for change include media visibility, legal actions, legislation and regulation, and research. Groups may work solo, in collaboration, or in coalition with other advocacy groups, with government and social services at the local, state, and national levels, and with health care services institutions. Foundations—including Villers, Robert Wood Johnson, W. Kellogg, and The California Endowment, support (or have supported) numerous community health advocacy efforts through financial and technical assistance.[73]

Given the diversity of community health advocacy groups, a meaningful analysis of them in relation to community justice is important, though necessarily general, as these groups have the potential to play many critical roles in fostering or frustrating community justice. Community health advocacy groups help communities effectively articulate their perspectives among others engaged in policy change, including health insurers, health care providers, health professional associations, and other community health advocacy groups. Each community within a given geographic health care community holds particular meanings and understandings about health and health care, and each has particular health care needs and priorities. The voices of all communities within the health care community are critical to the requisite diversity of perspectives for effective and just decision making.

Community justice requires that a just health care community recognize and respect all communities present within its boundaries. Some community health advocacy groups work to make health care policy more inclusive of marginalized or excluded communities: For example, Health Access California, a statewide coalition of health advocacy groups, including the California Immigrant Policy Center, was instrumental in mobilizing legislative and popular support for California's 2015 expansion of Medi-Cal (state Medicaid) coverage to all low-income California children, both documented and undocumented. These advocacy groups are working to recognize all California residents as members of a geographic (in this case, the state) health care community.

By and large, community health advocacy groups do not provide health care or public health services and, thus, are not directly responsible for the whole-person care required by community justice.[74] But some groups do advocate for particular health care services in the name of whole-person care. For example, many women's health organizations worked for ACA recognition of contraception as a preventive care service for women. Numerous local and state advocacy groups participate in a national health-equity movement that works to educate the public about the social determinants of health—namely, racism and poverty—and to build the recognition of "health in all policies." Such efforts require significant coalition building between advocacy groups and cross-sector work with public health and social services agencies, in particular around issues of housing, education, and food security.

Other advocacy groups work to "expos[e] prevailing norms and power relationships and mak[e] them available for public critique," as well as "seek to establish the legitimacy of different sorts of bodies or bodily experiences."[75] In her keynote speech at the 2014 Philadelphia Trans-Health Conference, Harper Jean Tobin laid out a plan for the future of the trans movement, leading with "the premise that there is nothing wrong with trans people, and we belong everywhere. . . . One of the most critical things we must stand for as a movement, together with many other movements, is that, to quote the performance artist Glenn Marla, 'there is no wrong way to have a body.' . . . Changing the law is only going to mean so much if we don't create the support, *in our local communities*, to make it real."[76] Some groups seek recognition and care for persons with stigmatized conditions such as mental illness; others for persons with "illnesses you have to fight to get" such as fibromyalgia.[77] Groups that work to reduce or eliminate fragmented health care practices, as well as those that attempt to expand the range of health-promoting practices and accessible practitioners, are advancing the whole-person care requisite for community justice.

Community health advocacy groups have their greatest potential community justice impact—and challenge—in relation to the third standard of health justice: participation as effective voice. As Roland Labonte asks, "How does one go about including individuals and groups in a set of structured social relationships responsible for excluding them in the first place?"[78] Indeed, as Iris Marion Young advises, societies with structural inequalities are likely to need advocacy and activism in addition to deliberative democracy to achieve justice.[79] Most advocacy groups are established precisely to strengthen a community's presence and voice about a particular health concern as well as to influence related policy. The sheer existence of these groups indicates that not all communities have voice or that some communities have voice but are not heard. In the name of community justice, how can we bring all communities to the health care decision-making table that has had seats for some but not all? How do we make it a "welcome table," which, in Bryan Massingale's words, is "the polar opposite of exclusion and neglect?"[80] Community justice requires that the health care table be enlarged and redesigned so that all can come to it with effective voice. How might community health advocacy groups help create the conditions for effective voice, that is, for diverse speech, respectful listening, dialogue, and understanding?

As noted earlier, advocacy groups use many different community organizing strategies for building participation: the Texas Latina Advocacy Network, part of the National Latina Institute for Reproductive Health, has focused attention on south Texas, where reproductive health services are scarce, distant, and declining. It has organized local communities in letter writing, marches, public hearings, and meetings with elected officials.[81] Forward Together, formerly Asian Communities for Reproductive Justice, has widened into a multiracial organization that recognizes that "reproductive justice is deeply tied to social, economic, and racial justice, and to work for one requires the vision and leadership to connect them all."[82] As such, Forward Together focuses on leadership development and cross-sector networking to create strong voices, particularly in support of strong families.

Paradoxically, invisibility can signal either a community's marginalization or its dominance—dominance being the uncritical normativity and privilege granted to, for example, the biomedical community or to the white community. Marginalization and dominance are interrelated, and both stand as obstacles to community justice. As Labonte puts it, "Our concern . . . should not be [only] with the groups or conditions that are excluded, but [also] with the socioeconomic rules and political powers that create excluded groups and conditions, and the social groups who benefit by this."[83]

Some community health organizing efforts intentionally focus on the relatively privileged and powerful, for example, to promote critical self-reflection as a means to recognize one's own values, assumptions, oppressions, and privileges.[84] Cheryl A. Hyde recommends a process of cultural self-assessment, especially for members of privileged groups whose perspectives have been granted a normativity that obscures their particularity.[85] This deeper self-understanding of one's cultural identity is key to recognizing privilege and developing relationships and communities capable of effective voice. Similarly, Galen Ellis and Sheryl Walton call for cultural humility rather than cultural competency, humility being "the ability to listen both to persons from other cultures and to our own internal dialogue. When we do that, we discover how easily we discount another's truth when it passes through our own cultural lens."[86]

Another promising advocacy effort for effective voice involves community building: a long-term approach that starts not with a particular health issue or policy but with assessing a community's strengths and then building community capacities.[87] For example, The California Endowment (TCE), in its Building Healthy Communities program, has come to understand that both "race and place matter." Says Anthony Iton, the senior vice president of TCE's Healthy Communities program, "To focus only on policy change is a subtly racist argument and ignores the fact of systemic devaluation of certain populations and the exclusion of those populations in the decisionmaking venues. . . . If we don't change power dynamics, political, economic, etc., just having those new policies is not going to make a difference. . . . The design [of Healthy Communities] shifted to a deeper investment of power building and lighter touch on prescriptive policy change. Now TCE sees policy change as a measure of change in community power."[88]

We do not know how well different community health advocacy efforts would actually facilitate participation as effective voice, but two recent evaluations of state consumer advocacy networks show that such networks do strengthen the effective advocacy of consumer groups. One evaluation assessed the Robert Wood Johnson Foundation's Consumer Voices for Coverage program, which supported a dozen state-based consumer advocacy organizations, each of which worked with a network of consumer groups within their state.[89] This appraisal found that the "program established collaborative networks and strengthened consumer advocates' capacities, leading to increases in their involvement and influence in shaping health coverage policy debates in their states."[90] Similarly an assessment of California Healthy Cities and Communities (CHCC) program, funded by The California Endowment, reports that "overall the CHCC coalitions were successful in engaging residents, either as coalition members, as participants in a community assessment, or participants in the coalition's implementation activities."[91] These efforts suggest that community health advocacy groups can play a critical role in fostering participation as effective voice.

Community health centers, community health needs assessments, and health advocacy groups already play significant roles in U.S. health care and health policy. These institutions, policies, and groups embody all three elements of community justice, even if partially, and thus constitute openings for the further development of community justice.

Conclusion

Health care as a community good is a health policy reality, and communities are necessary moral participants in theories of justice for health care. Community health centers, hospital community needs assessments, and community-based advocacy groups are among the more substantial and apparent expressions of community in U.S. health care. In and through these efforts multiple and diverse communities create critical meanings and understandings related to health and health care, shape health via their physical and social environments, care for the health needs of their sick and well residents, and receive the benefits of health care beyond improvements in individual health. Having explored some of the ways that these community health endeavors might promote or limit community justice, I conclude by integrating these policy insights and pointing to potential next steps for developing community justice in the making.

The health care community of community justice—geographically defined, inclusive of all residents, and constituted by many diverse (sub) communities—is only partially approached in current health policy efforts. While, technically speaking, community health centers (CHCs) and nonprofit hospitals could serve all residents in geographically defined areas, in usual practice, each serves more limited groups. The communities of CHCs are geographically defined but must also meet federally designated medically underserved area criteria that, in effect, privilege certain types of medical need over others. While patient populations of nonprofit hospitals typically have a geographic dimension to them, they generally do not include all community residents, as evidenced by their community benefit focus on financial assistance to individual patients rather than on community-wide health improvement efforts. Also the Internal Revenue Service (IRS)–mandated inclusion of medically underserved, low-income, and minority groups in the community health needs assessment (CHNA) process can reasonably be understood as a response to past and present exclusion of these groups. Numerous health advocacy groups work to make visible, and give voice to, those and other communities within local communities and states. Furthermore, neither CHCs nor nonprofit hospitals are sufficiently numerous to have geographic coverage over the entire nation and thus be inclusive of all U.S. residents.

Community justice requires that we create new health care communities, ones that are geographically defined, inclusive, internally diverse, interdependent, and that collectively provide nationwide coverage. Ultimately these just health care communities will require a national commitment to the respectful health care of all residents. Given current social and health care inequities, this inclusivity will also require additional resources to support the care of previously excluded groups and communities. One strategy building on current arrangements and working toward inclusive geographic communities could be to expand the current medically underserved area and population group criteria for community health centers to enable them to serve wider geographic areas and, thus, more and different residents. Another strategy could be to hold nonprofit hospitals accountable for defining their communities as inclusive of all residents in a designated geographic area, at least for community benefit and IRS tax-exemption purposes. Hospitals could also be held accountable for genuinely inclusive and participatory CHNA processes as well as for progress toward defined implementation goals. Hospitals could engage the health advocacy groups in their communities to help them identify particular communities so communities themselves could articulate their particular needs. These new more inclusive health care communities would build new interpersonal and institutional bonds and relations within and between communities and would be likely to produce community benefits extending beyond the health care realm.

In community justice it is the work of inclusive geographic communities to determine the precise nature of the health care to be offered in their communities, that is, within the bounds of just care understood broadly as care for whole persons both sick and well. While many health centers offer a relatively wide range of primary-care services and hospitals tend to offer more specialty care, patients of both institutions would benefit from greater attention to their particular social, relational, and cultural contexts and needs. Just care requires health care providers to engage in ongoing communication with their patients and other community members in order to appreciate their particular understandings of health, illness, and healing and thus to realize and respect their particular health care needs. Just care calls for culturally informed health care workers who interact well together in assessing and respecting their patients' particularities. In addition to more professionals, more community health workers, translators, and patient advocates would be needed. Innovative and more relational organizational structures for health care would be in order as well—for example, nurse practitioner clinics offering primary-care services and hospices for end-of-life care. Some Patient Protection and Affordable Care Act–prompted organizational and financing reforms currently under way seek greater coordination among health care providers and could potentially expand whole-person sick care across primary-care, specialty, mental, and behavioral health services. Notably, though, some national reforms simultaneously risk stripping away the specificity of community-based needs and priorities.

Just care must also attend to well-person care, for example, individual preventive health services and broader community-based health improvement activities. This community wellness orientation would require a significant cultural and structural reorientation by most health care practitioners and institutions in order to address, for example, the social inequities embedded in the social determinants of health, that is, in the economic, social, political, and environmental relations and institutions that affect health. To varying degrees, CHCs have attempted to address some of these social inequities, but a more concerted effort in addressing unhealthy community conditions is needed by these and other health care providers.

The CHNA is also a potential contribution toward just care as it requires that hospitals look beyond their patient populations to the nature of care needed by the wider community. Given that the primary focus of most hospitals is on the provision of personal sick care services and that the primary mission of public health and some community leaders is to improve the health of the community, just care suggests that hospitals should cooperate with and even follow the lead of public health and community leaders in identifying and responding to the social conditions that influence community health. The strengthening of community health improvement activities by nonprofit hospitals is supported by the IRS's approval of related expenses as community benefit expenditures. Just care as a norm of community justice would urge the IRS to allow or even to promote community benefit expenditures on community-building activities, thus incentivizing a wide array of community organizing and leadership development activities. Such resources might directly support the work of community health advocacy groups in bolstering their communities' understandings and articulations of their needs for both sick and well care. Health care providers and institutions could also support such community-building efforts, regardless of the IRS designation regarding allowable related expenses.

Just participation in community justice means that all community members are enabled to participate with effective voices in community decision making about health care. The governing boards of community health centers are a strong mechanism for community voices, and they sit in stark contrast to the weak community input of CHNAs. Effective voice would call for sustaining and strengthening CHC board governance and for reconfiguring the CHNA process, particularly in this era of institutional integration and policy reform. In community justice, all understandings of health and health care present in the health care community are important to the determination of the community's health care needs, priorities, and institutions. All communities within the geographic health care community must be regarded as important meaning makers who contribute to strong deliberation and thus are critical to community decision making.

Effective voice requires creating new institutional structures for democratic community participation. The more formal democratic deliberative processes—such as elected boards, commissions, and advisory boards—would be stronger if all community members had access to them. Given current social and political inequities, it is likely that such access will require the designation of some seats to specific communities that historically have been less heard within the larger health care community. Advocacy groups have a particularly important role to play in leadership development for such positions and in holding such democratic deliberative processes accountable to being fully inclusive. These institutional efforts must enable sustained discussions over time and cannot be single public deliberation events. Community engagement processes, created by all interested community members, would be put in place that facilitate new and optimally more inclusive ways of relating, including the sharing of community and individual narratives and novel meeting arrangements to accommodate the needs of all community members. Increased community participation with effective voices in deliberative health care decision making would likely build the self-respect and mutual respect of all involved, and thus they are likely to boost participation in other political realms of the community—a significant community benefit.

Past and present inequities in participation, power, attention, and voice in health care decision making mean that just participation as effective voice will necessitate somewhat differing roles and responsibilities for different groups (largely differing by degree). For relatively powerful and vocal groups or communities who are accustomed to speaking and to being heard, the participatory challenge would be to listen, seriously attend to, and understand perspectives unlike one's own in the name of recognizing and respecting diversity within the health care community. Effective voice requires not only listening but also a commitment by listeners to reconsider their own positions in light of the views of other community members. In a community justice framework, dominant communities would work to recognize their own particularities—including their gender, race, class, educational, and other privileges that mask or obscure other community voices—and privileges that set themselves up to be "the non-defined definers of other people."[1] This work toward effective voice is, in one sense, about "respect-ability," that is, the ability to respect—to attend perceptively to, and not to ignore or dismiss, the inherent moral value of all persons, all community members.

For relatively powerless groups and communities unaccustomed to speaking and being heard, the participatory challenge would be to strengthen voices that have been weakened or lost owing to oppression or unjust conditions. Achieving effective voice would likely involve long-term financial and other support for community organizing, community building, and advocacy efforts including leadership development. Given past and present inequities in participation, relatively powerless, nondominant communities must be engaged participants in health care deliberations from the start, rather than included after the leadership, rules of engagement, and agenda have been determined.

As becomes clear in this integration of policy insights, the fulfillment of one community justice norm is intricately tied to the fulfillment of the other two: effective voice in decision making, for example, requires that persons are recognized as community members, and the nature of whole-person care is determined largely by community participation in decision making. Also, the interdependence of the national and community levels of health care and health policy is apparent: The establishment of geographic and inclusive health care communities would likely be the result of a national commitment to the inclusion of all persons through this community mechanism, and the proposed provision of tertiary care at the national level enables more localized communities to focus on the more relational care. Such interconnections suggest not only policy complexity but also the multiplicity of potential sites for the cultivation of community justice.

In community justice, health care communities speak, hear, consider, question, discuss, and ultimately agree on particular understandings of health care based on the diverse understandings of health and health care within the community. Notably, community justice does not tell communities how to understand or value health and health care (beyond requiring care for the whole person) but, rather, opens up space in both justice theory and in health policy for thinking anew about just health care. This vision insists on the importance of communities through its fundamental understanding of health care as, in important part, a community good. Further serious consideration of communities as critical moral participants in the creation and praxis of just health care is needed in both the health policy and ethical realms.

Ultimately community justice in health care is about respect: the perceptive and attentive caring for all persons in their communities, each with their particular and equal moral value and worth. Community justice means respecting communities, including the diverse ways that they create and give meaning to health and health care and the agreements that they come to regarding health care. Finally, community justice calls us to re-spect, to look again, at how we understand justice in health care and at how we include communities, for only with them is respectful and just health care possible.

Notes

Introduction

1. Heather Widdows and Sean Cordell, "Why Communities and Their Goods Matter: Illustrated with the Example of Biobanks," *Public Health Ethics* 4, no. 1 (2011): 23.
2. Roland Labonte, "Social Inclusion/Exclusion: Dancing the Dialectic," *Health Promotion International* 19, no. 1 (March 1, 2004): 115–121, doi:10.1093/heapro/dah112.
3. Emilie Maureen Townes, *Womanist Ethics and the Cultural Production of Evil* (New York: Palgrave Macmillan, 2006), 137.
4. Michael Walzer, *Spheres of Justice: A Defense of Pluralism and Equality* (New York: Basic Books, 1983), 5.
5. Iris Marion Young, *Justice and the Politics of Difference* (Princeton, NJ: Princeton University Press, 1990), 5; emphasis in original.

Chapter 1 — Health Care as a Community Good

I thank the following for permission to reprint the epigraph: Jon P. Gunnemann, "Justice and the Good of Health," Church and Society, no. 4 (1989): 33. Reprinted by permission of the publisher.

1. David M. Craig, *Health Care as a Social Good: Religious Values and American Democracy* (Washington, DC: Georgetown University Press, 2014). Craig calls for greater recognition of health care as a social good and identifies its social dimensions as national: "Americans built US health care as a social good by pooling shared resources and responding to common vulnerability" (90). That said, Craig also attends to the actual and potential contributions of religious, largely Christian, communities and values in health care and health policy.
2. Michael L. Gross, "Speaking in One Voice or Many? The Language of Community," *Cambridge Quarterly of Health Care Ethics* 13 (January 1, 2004): 28, 32.
3. Ibid., 33.
4. Susan M. Wolf, ed., *Feminism and Bioethics: Beyond Reproduction* (New York: Oxford University Press, 1996).
5. John B. Cobb, Jr., "Defining Normative Community," in *Rooted in the Land: Essays on Community and Place*, ed. William Vitek and Wes Jackson (New Haven, CT: Yale University Press, 1996), 189.
6. Philip Selznick, *The Moral Commonwealth: Social Theory and the Promise of Community* (Berkeley: University of California Press, 1992), 358.
7. The bus example comes from Iris Marion Young's discussion of Jean-Paul Sartre's distinction between a group and a series (or serial collectivity). Neither Young nor Sartre would consider those waiting for a bus to be a community, though this series has the "latent potential" to become a group. Iris Marion Young, "Gender as Seriality: Thinking about Gender as a Social Collective," in *Intersecting Voices: Dilemmas of Gender, Political Philosophy, and Policy* (Princeton, NJ: Princeton University Press, 1997), 24.
8. Cobb, "Defining Normative Community," 189.

9. Kathleen M. MacQueen et al., "What Is Community? An Evidence-Based Definition for Participatory Public Health," *American Journal of Public Health* 91, no. 12 (December 2001): 1929–1938, quoted at 1929. Emphasis in original.

10. "Community," *OED Online* (Oxford: Oxford University Press, March 2012).

11. Elizabeth Frazer and Nicola Lacey, *The Politics of Community: A Feminist Critique of the Liberal-Communitarian Debate* (Toronto: University of Toronto Press, 1993), 202.

12. Rachel Jewkes and Anne Murcott, "Meanings of Community," *Social Science and Medicine* 43, no. 4 (August 1996): 555–563, doi:10.1016/0277–9536(95)00439–4.

13. Paul Starr, *The Social Transformation of American Medicine* (New York: Basic Books, 1982).

14. Elliot G. Mishler, "Viewpoint: Critical Perspectives on the Biomedical Model," in *Social Contexts of Health, Illness, and Patient Care*, ed. Elliot G. Mishler et al. (New York: Cambridge University Press, 1981), 1–23.

15. Elizabeth Fee and Nancy Krieger, "Understanding AIDS: Historical Interpretations and the Limits of Biomedical Individualism," *American Journal of Public Health* 83, no. 10 (October 1993): 1481.

16. Lynn Payer, *Medicine and Culture: Varieties of Treatment in the United States, England, West Germany, and France* (New York: Henry Holt, 1996).

17. Atul Gawande, "The Cost Conundrum," *New Yorker*, June 1, 2009, http://www.newyorker.com/reporting/2009/06/01/090601fa_fact_gawande?printable=true&currentPage=all.

18. Dartmouth Medical School and Center for the Evaluative Clinical Sciences, *The Dartmouth Atlas of Health Care, 1996* ([Chicago]: AHA Press, 1996), 2.

19. Mishler, "Viewpoint," 1 (italics in original).

20. Eliot Freidson, *Profession of Medicine: A Study of the Sociology of Applied Knowledge* (New York: Harper & Row, 1970), 206. "Epistemic community" is Burkart Holzner's term, quoted by Freidson, 206.

21. Peter Conrad, *The Medicalization of Society: On the Transformation of Human Conditions into Treatable Disorders* (Baltimore: Johns Hopkins University Press, 2007).

22. In this passage, Airhihenbuwa refers to allopathic hegemony in Africa, though I find that his trenchant critique of biomedicine transcends that continent and is apt for the United States. Collins O. Airhihenbuwa, *Health and Culture: Beyond the Western Paradigm* (Thousand Oaks, CA: Sage, 1995), 48.

23. Linda L. Barnes and Susan Starr Sered, eds., *Religion and Healing in America* (Oxford: New York: Oxford University Press, 2005).

24. Joseph D. Calabrese, *A Different Medicine: Postcolonial Healing in the Native American Church*, Oxford Ritual Studies (New York: Oxford University Press, 2013).

25. Wende Elizabeth Marshall, "Tasting Earth: Healing, Resistance Knowledge, and the Challenge to Dominion," *Anthropology and Humanism* 37, no. 1 (2012): 84–99, doi:10.1111/j.1548–1409.2012.01109.x.

26. Linda L. Barnes, "Multiple Meanings of Chinese Healing in the United States," in *Religion and Healing in America*, ed. Linda L. Barnes and Susan Starr Sered (Oxford and New York: Oxford University Press, 2005), 307–331.

27. Stephanie Y. Mitchem and Emilie Maureen Townes, eds., *Faith, Health, and Healing in African American Life,* Religion, Health, and Healing (Westport, CT, and London: Praeger, 2008).

28. Emilie Maureen Townes, *Breaking the Fine Rain of Death: African American Health Issues and a Womanist Ethic of Care* (New York: Continuum, 1998), 50.

29. Boston University School of Medicine, Graduate Medical Sciences, "Our Roots: The Boston Healing Landscape Project," n.d., http://www.bumc.bu.edu/gms/maccp/about/our-roots-the-boston-healing-landscape-project, accessed April 8, 2016.

30. Robert Peel, *Health and Medicine in the Christian Science Tradition: Principle, Practice, and Challenge* (New York: Crossroad, 1988); Mary Baker Eddy, *Science and Health, with Key to the Scriptures* (Boston: First Church of Christ, Scientist, 1971); Rennie B. Schoepflin, *Christian Science on Trial: Religious Healing in America* (Baltimore: Johns Hopkins University Press, 2002).

31. Anne Fadiman, *The Spirit Catches You and You Fall Down: A Hmong Child, Her American Doctors, and the Collision of Two Cultures*, 1st ed. (New York: Farrar, Straus, & Giroux, 1997).

32. Lori Arviso Alvord and Elizabeth Cohen, *The Scalpel and the Silver Bear* (New York: Bantam Books, 1999).

33. Everett R. Rhoades, *American Indian Health Innovations in Health Care, Promotion, and Policy* (Baltimore: Johns Hopkins University Press, 2000).

34. Steven Cummins et al., "Understanding and Representing 'Place' in Health Research: A Relational Approach," *Social Science and Medicine*, special issue: "Placing Health in Context," 65, no. 9 (November 2007): 1825, doi:10.1016/j.socscimed.2007.05.036; emphases in original.

35. Paula Braveman, Susan Egerter, and David R. Williams, "The Social Determinants of Health: Coming of Age," *Annual Review of Public Health* 32, no. 1 (March 18, 2011): 381–398, doi:10.1146/annurev-publhealth-031210-101218; Lisa F. Berkman and Ichiro Kawachi, *Social Epidemiology* (New York: Oxford University Press, 2000); Ichiro Kawachi, "Social Epidemiology," *Social Science and Medicine* 54, no. 12 (June 2002): 1739–1741, doi:10.1016/S0277–9536(01)00144–7.

36. David R. Williams et al., "Race, Socioeconomic Status, and Health: Complexities, Ongoing Challenges, and Research Opportunities," in *The Biology of Disadvantage: Socioeconomic Status and Health*, ed. Nancy E. Adler and Judith Stewart (Boston: Blackwell, on behalf of the New York Academy of Sciences, 2010).

37. Anna F. Abraido-Lanza, Maria T. Chao, and Karen R. Florez, "Do Healthy Behaviors Decline with Greater Acculturation? Implications for the Latino Mortality Paradox," *Social Science and Medicine* 61, no. 6 (September 2005): 1243–1255, doi:10.1016/j.socscimed.2005.01.016.

38. Frank W. Young and Thomas A. Lyson, "Structural Pluralism and All-Cause Mortality," *American Journal of Public Health* 91, no. 1 (January 2001): 136.

39. Ichiro Kawachi, "The Relationship between Health Assets, Social Capital, and Cohesive Communities," in *Health Assets in a Global Context*, ed. Antony Morgan, Maggie Davies, and Erio Ziglio (New York: Springer, 2010), 167–179.

40. Linda M. Burton et al., eds., *Communities, Neighborhoods, and Health: Expanding the Boundaries of Place*, vol. 1: *Social Disparities in Health and Health Care* (New York and London: Springer, 2011), vii.

41. Daniel Callahan, *What Kind of Life? The Limits of Medical Progress* (New York: Simon & Schuster, 1990), 144.

42. Lindsay Abrams, "Kind Neighbors Are Scarce, but Important," survey conducted for the *Atlantic* in conjunction with GlaxoSmithKline, March 6, 2013, http://www.theatlantic.com/health/archive/2013/03/kind-neighbors-are-scarce-but-important/273375/.

43. Mark Schlesinger, "Paradigms Lost: The Persisting Search for Community in U.S. Health Policy," *Journal of Health Politics, Policy, and Law* 22, no. 4 (August 1, 1997): 937–992, doi:10.1215/03616878–22–4-937.

44. Virginia M. Brennan, *Free Clinics: Local Responses to Health Care Needs* (Baltimore: Johns Hopkins University Press, 2013). Jennifer Nelson, *More than Medicine: A History of the Feminist Women's Health Movement* (New York: NYU Press, 2015). Alondra Nelson, *Body and Soul: The Black Panther Party and the Fight against Medical Discrimination* (Minneapolis: University of Minnesota Press, 2011).

45. Robert A. Scott et al., "Organizational Aspects of Caring," *Milbank Quarterly* 73, no. 1 (January 1, 1995): 81, 80, doi:10.2307/3350314.

46. Marc A. Rodwin, "The Neglected Remedy: Strengthening Consumer Voice in Managed Care," *American Prospect* 34 (October 1997): 45–51.

47. Peter Aggleton and Richard Parker, "Moving beyond Biomedicalization in the HIV Response: Implications for Community Involvement and Community Leadership among Men Who Have Sex with Men and Transgender People," *American Journal of Public Health* 105, no. 8 (August 2015): 1552–1558, doi:10.2105/AJPH.2015.302614.

48. Suzanne J. Crawford O'Brien, ed., *Religion and Healing in Native America: Pathways for Renewal*, Religion, Health, and Healing (Westport, CT: Praeger, 2008).

49. David Zuckerman, "Hospitals Building Healthier Communities: Embracing the Anchor Mission" (Takoma Park, MD: Democracy Collaborative at the University of Maryland, March 2013), 1, http://community-wealth.org/sites/clone.community -wealth.org/files/downloads/Zuckerman-HBHC-2013.pdf.

50. Dionne Searcey, "Hospitals Provide a Pulse in Struggling Rural Towns," Economy: A Shifting Middle, *New York Times*, April 29, 2015, http://www.nytimes .com/2015/04/30/business/economy/hospitals-provide-a-pulse-in-struggling-rural -towns.html.

Chapter 2 — Communities Obscured

1. The analysis of these six theories is not representative or comprehensive of all theories of justice in health care, but it does identify salient communities and their moral roles for this set of prominent justice theories in health care. Given the overlapping assumptions and norms across some of these theories, specific features of my analysis related to one theory may be relevant to other theories regardless of their categorization as either an egalitarian or a capability theory.

2. Norman Daniels, *Just Health: Meeting Health Needs Fairly* (Cambridge and New York: Cambridge University Press, 2008). Leonard M. Fleck, *Just Caring: Health Care Rationing and Democratic Deliberation* (Oxford and New York: Oxford University Press, 2009). Shlomi Segall, *Health, Luck, and Justice* (Princeton, NJ: Princeton University Press, 2009).

3. Daniels, *Just Health*, 1.

4. Ibid., 101.

5. Ibid., 117.

6. Ibid., 19, 211, 297.

7. Ibid., 52, 89–92, 299–301.

8. Ibid., 306.

9. Ibid., 22.

10. Ibid., 52.

11. Ibid., 113.
12. Ibid., 125.
13. Ibid., 124.
14. Ibid., 118.
15. Ibid., 30n1, emphasis added.
16. Michael Walzer, *Spheres of Justice: A Defense of Pluralism and Equality* (New York: Basic Books, 1983), 14n3.
17. Daniels, *Just Health*, 14.
18. Ibid., 346.
19. Ibid.
20. Ibid., 348.
21. Fleck, *Just Caring*, 140.
22. Ibid., 163.
23. Ibid., 34.
24. Ibid., 128.
25. Ibid., 163.
26. Ibid., 352–354.
27. Ibid., 192 (emphasis in original).
28. Ibid., 192–193.
29. Ibid., 360.
30. Ibid., 200; Vence L. Bonham et al., "Community-Based Dialogue: Engaging Communities of Color in the United States' Genetics Policy Conversation," *Journal of Health Politics, Policy and Law* 34, no. 3 (June 1, 2009): 325–359, doi:10.1215/03616878–2009–009.
31. Fleck, *Just Caring*, 200.
32. Ibid., 377.
33. Ibid., 163.
34. Segall, *Health, Luck, and Justice*.
35. Ibid., 141.
36. Ibid., 143.
37. Ibid., 209n16.
38. Ibid., 143.
39. Ibid., 144.
40. Ibid., 145.
41. Ibid., 144–148.
42. Ibid., 147.
43. Jennifer Prah Ruger, *Health and Social Justice* (Oxford and New York: Oxford University Press, 2010).
44. Sridhar Venkatapuram, *Health Justice: An Argument from the Capabilities Approach* (Cambridge: Polity, 2011). Madison Powers and Ruth R. Faden, *Social Justice: The Moral Foundations of Public Health and Health Policy*, Issues in Biomedical Ethics (Oxford and New York: Oxford University Press, 2006).
45. Ruger, *Health and Social Justice*, xi.
46. Ibid., 43.
47. Ibid., 154–155.
48. Ibid., xv.
49. Ibid., 16, 231, 207.
50. Ibid., 148–150.

51. Ibid., 116.
52. Ibid., 221.
53. Venkatapuram, *Health Justice*, 19.
54. Ibid., 23.
55. Ibid., 13.
56. Ibid., 210.
57. Ibid., 214.
58. Powers and Faden explain that their theory "has many affinities with and owes a considerable intellectual debt to capabilities theories," but "for a variety of reasons," they chose different terminology to describe their work. Powers and Faden, *Social Justice*, 37. Given these affinities, I have placed their work with capabilities accounts in this chapter.
59. Ibid., 87.
60. Ibid.
61. Ibid., 88.
62. Ibid., 61.
63. Many communities receive even less attention: those characterized by illness, sexuality, age, and ability, for example.
64. Ibid., 87.
65. Karla F. C. Holloway, *Private Bodies, Public Texts: Race, Gender, and a Cultural Bioethics* (Durham, NC: Duke University Press, 2011).

Chapter 3 — Communities Constrained

1. Ezekiel J. Emanuel, *The Ends of Human Life: Medical Ethics in a Liberal Polity* (Cambridge, MA: Harvard University Press, 1991).
2. Ibid., 162.
3. Ibid., 236.
4. Ibid.
5. Ibid., 105–106, 108.
6. Ibid., 236.
7. Ibid., 167.
8. Ibid., 247.
9. Ibid., 225.
10. Ibid., 172, 198–204.
11. Ibid., 242.
12. Ibid., 157.
13. Ibid., 220.
14. Ibid., 239–240.
15. Ibid., 215.
16. Ibid., 179–180.
17. Ibid., 213.
18. Ibid.
19. Ibid., 174.
20. Ibid., 297n84.
21. Ibid., 174; see also 184.
22. Ibid., 167.
23. Ibid., 238–239.

24. Ibid., 196.
25. Ibid., 169.
26. Ibid., 242.
27. Ibid., 148.
28. Ibid., 230. In his general discussion of the motivations for participation in delib-eration, Emanuel makes a much stronger claim, declaring that "it is only through such deliberations that we can achieve political autonomy, develop distinctive human capacities, and contribute to an enduring world, a people and its poster-ity, which lives beyond our death" (160). Mirroring these goals of deliberation is Emanuel's vision of the person, who is "(1) autonomous, (2) with fully developed capacities, including those capacities that can only be fully developed through participation in democratic deliberation, and (3) who has transcended his [*sic*] contingent existence through participation in the shaping and sustaining of his [*sic*] community" (157).
29. Ibid., 148.
30. Ibid., 182–183.
31. Ibid., 207.
32. Ibid., 165.
33. Ibid., 179, 185, 192–193, 224.
34. Ibid., 210. Now, twenty-five years later, with more than 1,200 health centers in oper-ation, it is clear that health centers have not failed.
35. Ibid., 228–229.
36. Ibid., 228.
37. Ibid., 229.
38. Ibid., 246, emphasis added.
39. Ibid., 181.
40. Ibid., 231.
41. Ibid., 248.
42. Ibid., 183.
43. Ibid., 217.

Chapter 4 — Community Justice

I thank the following for permission to reprint the epigraph: Margaret Farley, "A Femi-nist Version of Respect for Persons," first published in the Journal of Feminist Studies in Religion *9, nos. 1 and 2 (Spring/Fall 1993): 198. Reprinted by permission of the author.*

1. The phrase comes from title of the book by Beverly Wildung Harrison, *Justice in the Making: Feminist Social Ethics*, ed. Elizabeth M. Bounds et al. (Louisville, KY: Westminster John Knox Press, 2004).
2. Ezekiel J. Emanuel, *The Ends of Human Life: Medical Ethics in a Liberal Polity* (Cambridge, MA: Harvard University Press, 1991), 178.
3. Harrison, *Justice in the Making*, 21.
4. Bryan N. Massingale, *Racial Justice and the Catholic Church* (Maryknoll, NY: Orbis Books, 2010), 143.
5. Ibid.
6. Nancy Fraser, *Scales of Justice: Reimagining Political Space in a Globalizing World*, New Directions in Critical Theory (New York: Columbia University Press, 2009), 61–63.

7. Juan Thompson, "'No Justice, No Respect': Why the Ferguson Riots Were Justified," *The Intercept*, December 1, 2014. https://firstlook.org/theintercept/2014/12/01/justice-respect-ferguson-riots-justified/.

8. Edward Kent, "Justice as Respect for Person," *Southern Journal of Philosophy* 6, no. 2 (1968): 70, doi:10.1111/j.2041–6962.1968.tb02028.x.

9. U.S. Department of Health, Education, and Welfare, Office of the Secretary, *The Belmont Report: Ethical Principles and Guidelines for the Protection of Human Subjects of Research*, DHEW Publication nos. (OS) 78–0013 and 78–0014 (Washington, DC: National Commission for the Protection of Human Subjects of Biomedical and Behavioral Research, April 18, 1978).

10. Larry Churchill, "Toward a More Robust Autonomy: Revising the Belmont Report," in *Belmont Revisited: Ethical Principles for Research on Human Subjects*, ed. James F. Childress, Eric M. Meslin, and Harold T. Shapiro (Washington, DC: Georgetown University Press, 2005), 117–118.

11. Margaret A. Farley, "A Feminist Version of Respect for Persons," *Journal of Feminist Studies in Religion* 9, nos. 1 and 2 (April 1, 1993): 187.

12. This recognition/appraisal typology as described by Stephen Darwall is one of many typologies of respect found in Robin S. Dillon, "Respect," in *The Stanford Encyclopedia of Philosophy*, ed. Edward N. Zalta, Spring 2014 ed., http://plato.stanford.edu/archives/spr2014/entries/respect/.

13. Susan Sherwin, "A Relational Approach to Autonomy in Health Care," in *The Politics of Women's Health: Exploring Agency and Autonomy*, by the Feminist Health Care Ethics Research Network, coord. Susan Sherwin (Philadelphia: Temple University Press, 1998); Farley, "A Feminist Version of Respect for Persons."

14. Karen Lebacqz, "We Sure Are Older But Are We Wiser?," in *Belmont Revisited: Ethical Principles for Research on Human Subjects*, ed. James F. Childress, Eric M. Meslin, and Harold T. Shapiro (Washington, DC: Georgetown University Press, 2005), 105.

15. Churchill, "Toward a More Robust Autonomy," 111–125.

16. Patricia A. King, "Justice beyond Belmont," in *Belmont Revisited: Ethical Principles for Research with Human Subjects*, ed. James F. Childress, Eric M. Meslin, and Harold T. Shapiro (Washington, DC: Georgetown University Press, 2005), 136–147.

17. This proposed principle of respect for communities has many of the same limitations as Emanuel's liberal-communitarian framework noted in chap. 3. See Ezekiel J. Emanuel and Charles Weijer, "Protecting Communities in Research: From a New Principle to Rational Protections," in *Belmont Revisited: Ethical Principles for Research with Human Subjects*, ed. James F. Childress, Eric M. Meslin, and Harold T. Shapiro (Washington, DC: Georgetown University Press, 2005), 165–183.

18. Lisa A. Eckenwiler, *Long-Term Care and Globalization: An Ecological Approach* (Baltimore: Johns Hopkins University Press, 2012), 84.

19. Larry L. Rasmussen, *Moral Fragments and Moral Community: A Proposal for Church in Society* (Minneapolis: Fortress Press, 1993), 125.

20. Robin S. Dillon, "Respect and Care: Toward Moral Integration," *Canadian Journal of Philosophy* 22, no. 1 (March 1992): 129.

21. Ibid., 122.

22. Farley, "A Feminist Version of Respect for Persons," 198.

23. Aretha Franklin, performer, "Respect," by Otis Redding, produced by Jerry Wexler and Arif Mardin, Atlantic Records, 1967.

24. My thanks to Irene Mata for drawing this temporal link.

25. Dillon, "Respect," *Stanford Encyclopedia*.

26. Ibid.

27. Michael Walzer, *Spheres of Justice: A Defense of Pluralism and Equality* (New York: Basic Books, 1983), 314; emphasis added.

28. Ibid., 28–29.

29. Ibid., 29.

30. Emanuel, *The Ends of Human Life*, 236.

31. These two criteria may conflict as operational feasibility of some services tends toward larger groupings while effective participation tends toward smaller groupings.

32. Arguably, a certain degree of relationality might be lost in making tertiary care a nationally defined and allocated good. It would also be possible to define tertiary care at the national level but to allow communities to control access to those services allocated to their district. For example, each district might decide who would receive certain services although the number of services available might be determined nationally.

33. Policy provisions would need to be made for persons without a clearly identifiable single or primary residence, for example, homeless persons, mobile populations such as migrant agricultural workers, and the multiresidenced affluent. A general residency criterion would likely need to be established to avoid persons having membership in multiple health care communities.

34. Institute of Medicine, *Improving Health in the Community: A Role for Performance Monitoring* (Washington, DC: National Academy Press, 1997), 25.

35. Peter Aggleton and Richard Parker, "Moving Beyond Biomedicalization in the HIV Response: Implications for Community Involvement and Community Leadership among Men Who Have Sex with Men and Transgender People," *American Journal of Public Health* 105, no. 8 (August 2015): 1552–1558, doi:10.2105/AJPH.2015.302614.

36. Jim Ife, *Community Development: Creating Community Alternatives—Vision, Analysis, and Practice* (Melbourne: Longman, 1995), 91.

37. Mark Schlesinger, "Paradigms Lost: The Persisting Search for Community in U.S. Health Policy," *Journal of Health Politics, Policy, and Law* 22, no. 4 (August 1, 1997): 937–992, doi:10.1215/03616878-22-4-937.

38. Paul Starr, *The Social Transformation of American Medicine* (New York: Basic Books, 1982); Charlene Galarneau, "Nineteenth-Century Religious Hospitals: Community and Communities" (unpublished paper, April 1, 1991), author's library.

39. Iris Marion Young, *Justice and the Politics of Difference* (Princeton, NJ: Princeton University Press, 1990), chap. 8; Marilyn Friedman, "Feminism and Modern Friendship: Dislocating the Community," *Ethics* 99, no. 2 (January 1989): 275–290.

40. Elizabeth Frazer and Nicola Lacey, *The Politics of Community: A Feminist Critique of the Liberal-Communitarian Debate* (Toronto: University of Toronto Press, 1993), 200. Emphasis in original.

41. Charlene Galarneau, "Still Missing: Undocumented Immigrants in Health Care Reform," *Journal of Health Care for the Poor and Underserved* 22, no. 2 (2011): 422–428, doi:10.1353/hpu.2011.0040.

42. National Immigration Law Center, "A Quick Guide to Immigrant Eligibility for ACA and Key Federal Means-Tested Programs, September 2015," *Access to Public Benefits—National Immigration Law Center*, https://www.nilc.org/wp-content/

uploads/2015/11/imm-eligibility-quickguide-2015–09–21.pdf, accessed April 2, 2016.

43. "Advocates: Extending Medi-Cal to Undocumented Kids a First Step," *California Healthline*, July 7, 2015, http://www.californiahealthline.org/articles/2015/7/7/advocates-extending-medical-to-undocumented-kids-a-good-first-step.

44. Rachana Pradhan, "California May Let Undocumented Immigrants Buy Obamacare," *POLITICO*, July 17, 2015, http://www.politico.com/story/2015/07/california-may-let-undocumented-immigrants-buy-obamacare-120249.html. In early September 2015, advocates for a federal waiver ended their effort, citing insufficient time in this legislative session to gather sufficient political support. See Judy Lin, "Sen. Ricardo Lara Drops Covered California Waiver for Immigrants," *Los Angeles Daily News*, September 4, 2015, http://www.dailynews.com/health/20150904/sen-ricardo-lara-drops-covered-california-waiver-for-immigrants.

45. "Tempers Flare as Huntington Park Appoints Undocumented Immigrants to City Commissions," CBS Los Angeles, August 4, 2015, http://losangeles.cbslocal.com/2015/08/04/tempers-flare-when-huntington-park-appoints-2-undocumented-immigrants-to-city-commissions/.

46. City of Huntington Park, California, "The Official Site of Huntington Park, CA!—Commissions," http://www.hpca.gov/index.aspx?nid=60, accessed August 12, 2015.

47. Daniel Callahan, *What Kind of Life? The Limits of Medical Progress* (New York: Simon & Schuster, 1990), 149.

48. Margaret A. Farley, *Compassionate Respect: A Feminist Approach to Medical Ethics and Other Questions*, 2002 Madeleva Lecture in Spirituality (New York: Paulist Press, 2002), 37–38.

49. Barbara Herman, "The Scope of Moral Requirement," *Philosophy and Public Affairs* 30, no. 3 (Summer 2001): 231.

50. Colleen T. Fogarty, "Call It 'Jiffy Boob': What's Lacking When Care Has Assembly-Line Efficiency," *Health Affairs* 30, no. 11 (November 1, 2011): 2206, doi:10.1377/hlthaff.2010.1106.

51. Eric J. Cassell, *The Healer's Art: A New Approach to the Doctor-Patient Relationship* (Philadelphia: Lippincott, 1976), 100.

52. Nadine J. Kaslow et al., "Health Care for the Whole Person: Research Update," *Professional Psychology: Research and Practice* 38, no. 3 (2007): 278–289; Tom A. Hutchinson, ed., *Whole Person Care: A New Paradigm for the 21st Century* (New York: Springer, 2011); Andrew Miles, "Towards a *Medicine of the Whole Person*—Knowledge, Practice, and Holism in the Care of the Sick," *Journal of Evaluation in Clinical Practice*, special issue: "Evidence Based Medicine" 15, no. 6 (December 2009): 941–949.

53. Miles, "Towards a *Medicine of the Whole Person*," 948.

54. Louise Aronson, "Necessary Steps: How Health Care Fails Older Patients, and How It Can Be Done Better," *Health Affairs* 34, no. 3 (March 1, 2015): 532, doi:10.1377/hlthaff.2014.1238.

55. Ibid., 530–531.

56. Cassell, *The Healer's Art*, 88–89, emphases in original.

57. Kaslow et al., "Health Care for the Whole Person."

58. Norma J. Peal and Francisco A. R. Garcia, "Interdisciplinary Models for Women's Health: A Literature Review," *Archives: The International Journal of Medicine* 2, no. 1 (January 2009): 211.

59. Lucian L. Leape et al., "Perspective: A Culture of Respect, Part 1: The Nature and Causes of Disrespectful Behavior by Physicians," *Academic Medicine: Journal of the Association of American Medical Colleges* 87, no. 7 (July 2012): 845–852, doi:10.1097/ACM.0b013e318258338d.

60. Ted J. Kaptchuk and David M. Eisenberg, "Varieties of Healing," *Annals of Internal Medicine* 135, no. 3 (August 7, 2001): part 1, "Medical Pluralism in the United States," 189–195, and part 2, "A Taxonomy of Unconventional Healing Practices," 196–204.

61. Structural competency is being knowledgeable about the structural contributions to health outcomes. See Jonathan M. Metzl and Helena Hansen, "Structural Competency: Theorizing a New Medical Engagement with Stigma and Inequality," *Social Science and Medicine*, special issue: "Structural Stigma and Population Health," 103 (February 2014): 126–133, doi:10.1016/j.socscimed.2013.06.032.

62. "Effective voice" appears in the works of various justice theorists, for example, David M. Smith, *Geography and Social Justice* (Oxford and Cambridge, MA: Blackwell, 1994), 293; and Young, *Justice and the Politics of Difference*, 251.

63. Lisa Sowle Cahill, *Theological Bioethics: Participation, Justice, and Change*, Moral Traditions Series (Washington, DC: Georgetown University Press, 2005), 43.

64. David Hollenbach, *Claims in Conflict: Retrieving and Renewing the Catholic Human Rights Tradition*, Woodstock Studies no. 4 (New York: Paulist Press, 1979), 152; emphasis in original.

65. J. Bryan Hehir, "Social Justice," in *The HarperCollins Encyclopedia of Catholicism*, ed. Richard P. McBrien and Harold W. Attridge (San Francisco: HarperSanFrancisco, 1995), 1204.

66. Young, *Justice and the Politics of Difference*, 92–93.

67. Fraser, *Scales of Justice*, 28–29.

68. Hollenbach, *Claims in Conflict*, 86.

69. Young, *Justice and the Politics of Difference*, 55.

70. Ibid., 91–95; Frazer and Lacey, *The Politics of Community*, 203–212; Susan Sherwin, *No Longer Patient: Feminist Ethics and Health Care* (Philadelphia: Temple University Press, 1992), 68–70.

71. Frazer and Lacey, *The Politics of Community*, 203.

72. Christopher F. Karpowitz, Tali Mendelberg, and Lee Shaker, "Gender Inequality in Deliberative Participation," *American Political Science Review* 106, no. 3 (August 2012): 533–547, doi:10.1017/S0003055412000329.

73. Rodriguez and colleagues find that excess Black deaths, like felony disenfranchisement, skew democratic political processes. See Javier M. Rodriguez et al., "Black Lives Matter: Differential Mortality and the Racial Composition of the U.S. Electorate, 1970–2004," *Social Science and Medicine* 136/137 (July 2015): 193–199, doi:10.1016/j.socscimed.2015.04.014.

74. Frazer and Lacey, *The Politics of Community*, 145.

75. John Stone, "Race and Healthcare Disparities: Overcoming Vulnerability," *Theoretical Medicine and Bioethics* 23, no. 6 (November 2002): 508, doi:10.1023/A:1021524431845.

76. Dillon, "Respect," *Stanford Encyclopedia*.

77. Sara Lawrence-Lightfoot, "Respect: On Witness and Justice," *American Journal of Orthopsychiatry* 82, no. 3 (July 2012): 454, doi:10.1111/j.1939–0025.2012.01174.x.

78. Iris Marion Young, "Asymmetrical Reciprocity: On Moral Respect, Wonder, and Enlarged Thought," in *Intersecting Voices: Dilemmas of Gender, Political Philosophy, and Policy* (Princeton, NJ: Princeton University Press, 1997), 56.
79. Ibid.
80. Ibid., 55.
81. Ibid., 56.
82. Ibid., 58.
83. The growing bioethical focus on public deliberation appears to be a notably different project than effective voice in community justice in that it attends largely to short-term, often onetime, events and exercises in which individuals discern their values and priorities about a given issue or proposal, often without an actual community context or within a hypothetical community. See Julia Abelson et al., "Public Deliberation in Health Policy and Bioethics: Mapping an Emerging, Interdisciplinary Field," *Journal of Public Deliberation* 9, no. 1 (April 30, 2013), http://www.publicdeliberation.net/jpd/vo19/iss1/art5; Erika Blacksher, "Participatory and Deliberative Practices in Health: Meanings, Distinctions, and Implications for Health Equity," *Journal of Public Deliberation* 9, no. 1 (April 30, 2013), http://www.publicdeliberation.net/jpd/vo19/iss1/art6; Erika Blacksher, Elizabeth Rigby, and Claire Espey, "Public Values, Health Inequality, and Alternative Notions of a 'Fair' Response," *Journal of Health Politics, Policy, and Law* 35, no. 6 (December 1, 2010): 889–920, doi:10.1215/03616878–2010–033; and several articles in *Hastings Center Report* 42, no. 2 (2012), doi:10.1002/hast.26.
84. Stone, "Race and Healthcare Disparities."
85. For vivid documentation and analysis of the individual, interpersonal, and institutional experiences of persons with chronic illness, see Sally E. Thorne, *Negotiating Health Care: The Social Context of Chronic Illness* (Newbury Park, CA: Sage, 1993).
86. Beatrix Rebecca Hoffman et al., eds., *Patients as Policy Actors*, Critical Issues in Health and Medicine (New Brunswick, NJ: Rutgers University Press, 2011); Steven Epstein, "Patient Groups and Health Movements," in *The Handbook of Science and Technology Studies*, ed. Edward J. Hackett et al., 3rd ed. (Cambridge, MA: MIT Press in cooperation with the Society for the Social Studies of Science, 2008), 499–539.
87. Iris Marion Young, "Activist Challenges to Deliberative Democracy," *Political Theory* 29, no. 5 (October 1, 2001): 670–690, doi:10.1177/0090591701029005004.
88. Ibid.

Chapter 5 — Community Justice in U.S. Health Policy

I thank the following for permission to reprint the epigraph: Deborah Stone, Policy Paradox: The Art of Political Decision Making, *3rd ed. (New York: W. W. Norton, 2012). Reprinted by permission of the publisher.*

1. Mark Schlesinger, "Paradigms Lost: The Persisting Search for Community in U.S. Health Policy," *Journal of Health Politics, Policy, and Law* 22, no. 4 (August 1, 1997): 937–992, doi:10.1215/03616878–22–4–937.
2. Accountable health communities are one reform effort that might hold promise for community justice, but they are too early in their development for a meaningful assessment. See Janet M. Corrigan and Elliott S. Fisher, "Accountable Health Communities: Insights from State Health Reform Initiatives" (Lebanon, NH: Dartmouth Institute for Health Policy and Clinical Practice, November 2014), http://tdi.dartmouth

.edu/research/evaluating/health-system-focus/accountable-care-organizations/
accountable-health-communities:-insights-from-state-health-reform-initiatives.

3. Charlene Galarneau, "Health Care Sharing Ministries and Their Exemption from the Individual Mandate of the Affordable Care Act," *Journal of Bioethical Inquiry* 12, no. 2 (February 12, 2015): 269–282, doi:10.1007/s11673–015–9610–3.

4. This historical sketch is drawn from the following works: Alice Sardell, *The U.S. Experiment in Social Medicine: The Community Health Center Program, 1965–1986* (Pittsburgh, PA: University of Pittsburgh Press, 1988); Isabel Marcus, *Dollars for Reform: The OEO Neighborhood Health Centers* (Lexington, MA: Lexington Books, 1981); Bonnie Lefkowitz, *Community Health Centers: A Movement and the People Who Made It Happen*, Critical Issues in Health and Medicine (New Brunswick, NJ: Rutgers University Press, 2007); and Jennifer Nelson, *More than Medicine: A History of the Feminist Women's Health Movement* (New York: NYU Press, 2015), chap. 1.

5. Sardell, *The U.S. Experiment in Social Medicine*, 52–53.

6. Marcus, *Dollars for Reform*, 6–7.

7. H. Jack Geiger, "Community Health Centers: Health Care as an Instrument of Social Change," in *Reforming Medicine: Lessons of the Last Quarter Century*, ed. Victor W. Sidel and Ruth Sidel (New York: Pantheon Books, 1984), 12–13. Simultaneously, Geiger and his vision were being challenged by other physician activists who believed that federal funding and outside involvement in neighborhood health centers could not lead to radical reform. For an analysis of this debate, see Jenna Loyd, "Where Is Community Health? Racism, the Clinic, and the Biopolitical State," in *Rebirth of the Clinic: Places and Agents in Contemporary Health Care*, ed. Cindy Patton (Minneapolis: University of Minnesota Press, 2010), 39–67.

8. Mildred A. Morehead, book review of *The U.S. Experiment in Social Medicine: The Community Health Center Program, 1965–1986*, by Alice Sardell, *Journal of Public Health Policy* 10, no. 2 (Summer 1989): 266, doi:10.2307/3342687.

9. Karen Davis and Cathy Schoen, *Health and the War on Poverty: A Ten-Year Appraisal* (Washington, DC: Brookings Institution, 1978).

10. Ibid., 163–173.

11. Sardell, *The U.S. Experiment in Social Medicine*, 106.

12. National Association of Community Health Centers, "Community Health Centers Past, Present, and Future: Building on 50 Years of Success," March 2015, http://www.nachc.com/client//PI_50th.pdf.

13. U.S. Department of Health and Human Services, Health Resources and Services Administration, "Health Center Program Terminology Tip Sheet," n.d., bphc.hrsa .gov/technicalassistance/healthcenterterminologysheet.pdf, accessed July 11, 2015.

14. Tribal clinics and Urban Indian Health Organizations are also eligible for FQHC certification, but the federal Health Resources and Services Administration does not administer these programs.

15. Calling a community health center an "FQHC" oddly refers to a health center by a single financial characteristic, that is, its certification status for a particular level of Medicare and Medicaid reimbursement. Notably, in 2013, only 49.9 percent of grantee center patients were beneficiaries of Medicare or Medicaid. See U.S. Department of Health and Human Services, Health Resources and Services Administration, "2013 Health Center Data: National Program Grantee Data," http://bphc.hrsa.gov/uds/datacenter.aspx, accessed July 11, 2015. This naming convention may reflect an increasing financial framing of all health care institutions. I use "FQHCs" only when

CMS designation is relevant. Otherwise I use the legislative terms "community health centers" to refer to grantee health centers that serve all residents of a medically underserved area and "health centers" to represent all grantee health centers plus FQHC-LAs.

16. National Association of Community Health Centers, "United States Health Center Fact Sheet, 2013," 2014, https://www.nachc.com/client//United_States_FS_2014.pdf.

17. "2013 Health Center Data: National Program Grantee Data."

18. National Association of Community Health Centers, "Community Health Centers Past, Present, and Future."

19. Health centers are sometimes referred to as being a national network, but as community-based institutions, they function relatively independently of one another in day-to-day practice.

20. National Association of Community Health Centers, "Community Health Centers Past, Present, and Future."

21. Robert W. Mickey, "Dr. StrangeRove; or, How Conservatives Learned to Stop Worrying and Love Community Health Centers," in *The Health Care Safety Net in a Post-reform World*, ed. Sara Rosenbaum and Mark A. Hall (New Brunswick, NJ: Rutgers University Press, 2012), 55.

22. Peter Shin, Jessica Sharac, and Sara Rosenbaum, "Community Health Centers and Medicaid at 50: An Enduring Relationship Essential for Health System Transformation," *Health Affairs* 34, no. 7 (July 1, 2015): 1100, doi:10.1377/hlthaff.2015.0099.

23. Sara Rosenbaum, "Reinventing a Classic: Community Health Centers and the Newly Insured," in *The Health Care Safety Net in a Post-reform World*, ed. Mark A. Hall and Sara Rosenbaum (New Brunswick, NJ: Rutgers University Press, 2012), 67–90.

24. Mickey, "Dr. StrangeRove; or, How Conservatives Learned to Stop Worrying and Love Community Health Centers," 55.

25. U.S. Department of Health and Human Services, Health Resources and Services Administration, "Medically Underserved Areas/Populations: Guidelines for MUA and MUP Designation," June 1995, http://www.hrsa.gov/shortage/mua/index.html. Circumstances unaccounted for by these four variables may be factored into consideration of an "exceptional" MUP designation.

26. Barbara A. Cohen, "Re: Designation of People with Serious Mental Illnesses as a Special Medically Underserved Population," letter to Beth Rosenfeld, Health Resources and Services Administration, July 8, 2011, 4, http://www.hrsa.gov/advisorycommittees/shortage/Meetings/20111012/publiccommenthorizonhouse.pdf.

27. Fenway Institute et al., "The Case for Designating LGBT People as a Medically Underserved Population and as a Health Professional Shortage Area Population Group" (Boston: Fenway Institute, August 2014).

28. U.S. Department of Health and Human Services, Health Research and Services Administration, "Negotiated Rulemaking Committee on the Designation of Medically Underserved Populations and Health Professional Shortage Areas: Final Report to the Secretary" ("Final Report"), October 31, 2011, http://www.hrsa.gov/advisorycommittees/shortage/nrmcfinalreport.pdf.

29. Ibid., 15.

30. Ibid., 10.

31. As of July 10, 2015, the "Final Report" remains under review, according to Andy Jordan in an e-mail to the author.

32. U.S. Department of Health and Human Services, Health Research and Services Administration, "Final Report." In the proposed Index of Primary Care formula, the physician-to-provider ratio is more nuanced in that it counts only primary care physicians (not all physicians) and includes such nonphysician providers as physician assistants, nurse practitioners, and certified nurse midwives. The infant mortality rate component is replaced by two equally weighted indicators: the standardized mortality rate, and either the low birth weight rate or diabetes prevalence. The ability-to-pay component is expanded to 200 percent of the federal poverty level, and the age component is refashioned into a "barriers-to-care" (also called "risk factors") component, with five possible indicators, of which applicants choose two: percentage of the population who are (1) of "Hispanic ethnicity," (2) a "Racial Minority," (3) "with a Disability," (4) uninsured and under 400 percent of the poverty level, and (5) population density or travel time. Referring to Hispanics, racial minorities, disabled persons, and low-income, uninsured persons as "barriers to care" and "risk factors," no matter what percentage of the population they are, misrepresents and dehumanizes these groups, as well as obscures the actual barriers to care.

33. Rosy Chang Weir et al., "Use of Enabling Services by Asian American, Native Hawaiian, and Other Pacific Islander Patients at 4 Community Health Centers," *American Journal of Public Health* 100, no. 11 (November 2010): 2199–2205, doi:10.2105/AJPH.2009.172270.

34. Public Health and Welfare Act, 42 U.S.C. c. 6A(II)(D)(i): "Health Centers," 2015, Office of Law Revision Counsel: United States Code. http://uscode.house.gov/view.xhtml?path=/prelim@title42/chapter6A/subchapter2/partD/subpart1&edition=prelim.

35. Michelle Proser, "Deserving the Spotlight: Health Centers Provide High-Quality and Cost-Effective Care," *Journal of Ambulatory Care Management* 28, no. 4 (December 2005): 321–330.

36. Daren R. Anderson and J. Nwando Olayiwola, "Community Health Centers and the Patient-Centered Medical Home: Challenges and Opportunities to Reduce Health Care Disparities in America," *Journal of Health Care for the Poor and Underserved* 23, no. 3 (2012): 949–957.

37. Arshiya A. Baig et al., "Community Health Center Provider and Staff's Spanish Language Ability and Cultural Awareness," *Journal of Health Care for the Poor and Underserved* 25, no. 2 (2014): 527–545, doi:10.1353/hpu.2014.0086.

38. Ibid., 539.

39. Brian M. Shelley et al., "'They Don't Ask Me So I Don't Tell Them': Patient-Clinician Communication about Traditional, Complementary, and Alternative Medicine," *Annals of Family Medicine* 7, no. 2 (April 3, 2009): 139–147, doi:10.1370/afm.947. Sandra K. Burge and Teresa L. Albright, "Use of Complementary and Alternative Medicine among Family Practice Patients in South Texas," *American Journal of Public Health* 92, no. 10 (October 2002): 1614–1616.

40. National Association of Community Health Centers, "Health Centers Addressing the Social Determinants of Health: Protocol for Responding to and Assessing Patient Assets, Risks, and Experiences (PRAPARE)," February 2015, https://www.nachc.com/client/PRAPARE%20abstract%20%20LC%20overview%202%2026%2015.pdf.

41. National Association of Community Health Centers, "Going Beyond Primary Care: Health Centers Transform Health Care in Local Communities," 2013, https://www .nachc.com/client//Infographic_Final.pdf.

42. For a history and discussion of the debate over the use of the terms "patient" versus "consumer," see Nancy Tomes, "Patients or Health-Care Consumers? Why the History of Contested Terms Matters," in *History and Health Policy in the United States: Putting the Past Back In*, ed. Rosemary A. Stevens, Charles E. Rosenberg, and Lawton R. Burns (New Brunswick, NJ: Rutgers University Press, 2006), 83–110.

43. Public Health and Welfare Act, 42 U.S.C. c. 6A(II)(D)(i): "Health Centers."

44. U.S. Department of Health and Human Services Administration, Health Resources and Services Administration, "Health Center Program Governance," PIN 2014–01, January 27, 2014, http://bphc.hrsa.gov/programrequirements/policies/pin201401 .html.

45. Michael E. Samuels and Sudha Xirasagar, "National Survey of Community Health Centers Board Chairs" (Kansas City, MO: National Rural Health Association, May 2, 2005).

46. Brad Wright and Graham P. Martin, "Mission, Margin, and the Role of Consumer Governance in Decision Making at Community Health Centers," *Journal of Health Care for the Poor and Underserved* 25, no. 2 (2014): 930–947, doi:10.1353/ hpu.2014.0107.

47. Brad Wright, "Who Governs Federally Qualified Health Centers?" *Journal of Health Politics, Policy, and Law* 38, no. 1 (February 1, 2013): 27–55, doi:10.1215/03616878–1898794.

48. Patricia Fairchild and Pamela J. Byrnes, "Public Centers: A Discussion Monograph" (Bethesda, MD: National Association of Community Health Centers, April 2014), http://www.nachc.com/client/documents/2014PublicCentersMonograph.pdf.

49. Donna C. Folkemer et al., "Hospital Community Benefits after the ACA: The Emerging Federal Framework," Hospital Community Benefits Program (Baltimore: Hilltop Institute, University of Maryland, Baltimore County, January 2011), https://folio .iupui.edu/handle/10244/1011; Alice A. Noble and Andrew L. Hyams, "Charitable Hospital Accountability: A Review and Analysis of Legal and Policy Initiatives," *Journal of Law, Medicine and Ethics* 26, no. 2 (Summer 1998): 116; Stephen M. Shortell, Pamela K. Washington, and Raymond J. Baxter, "The Contribution of Hospitals and Health Care Systems to Community Health," *Annual Review of Public Health* 30, no. 1 (April 2009): 373–383, doi:10.1146/annurev.publhealth.032008.112750; Mark Schlesinger and Bradford Gray, "A Broader Vision for Managed Care, Part 1: Measuring the Benefit to Communities," *Health Affairs* 17, no. 3 (May 1, 1998): 152–168, doi:10.1377/hlthaff.17.3.152.

50. Quoting Gustafsson in Folkemer et al., "Hospital Community Benefits after the ACA," 2.

51. On various meanings of community benefits, see Mark Schlesinger et al., "A Broader Vision for Managed Care, Part 2: A Typology of Community Benefits," *Health Affairs* 17, no. 5 (September 1, 1998): 26–49, doi:10.1377/hlthaff.17.5.26.

52. Folkemer et al., "Hospital Community Benefits after the ACA," 2.

53. One could argue that care for some community members benefits the entire community, but this was not the direction taken. See Schlesinger et al., "A Broader Vision for Managed Care, Part 2," 29.

54. Noble and Hyams, "Charitable Hospital Accountability," 117.

55. Quoting Eric Weissenstein in ibid., 119.

56. Simone R. Singh et al., "Research and Practice. Analysis of Hospital Community Benefit Expenditures' Alignment with Community Health Needs: Evidence from a National Investigation of Tax-Exempt Hospitals," *American Journal of Public Health* 105, no. 5 (May 2015): 914–921, doi:10.2105/AJPH.2014.302436.

57. American Hospital Association, "Fast Facts on US Hospitals," 2014, http://www .aha.org/research/rc/stat-studies/fast-facts.shtml.

58. U.S. Department of Treasury, Internal Revenue Service, "Additional Requirement for Charitable Hospitals; Community Health Needs Assessments for Charitable Hospitals; Requirement of a Section 4959 Excise Tax Return and Time for Filing Return; Final Rule," *Federal Register* 79, no. 250 (December 31, 2014), 26 C.F.R. Parts 1, 53, and 602:78953–79016.

59. Ibid., 79002.

60. Ibid.

61. U.S. Department of Treasury, Internal Revenue Service, "Instructions for Schedule H (Form 990)," 2014, 4. Emphasis added.

62. Calling the IRS instructions "tentative," the American Hospital Association and the Catholic Hospital Association together have sought clarification, specifically citing housing improvements as a clear benefit to individual and community health. See Melina Reid Hatton and Lisa Gilden, letter to Ms. Sunita Lough, Commissioner, Tax Exempt and Government Entities Division, Internal Revenue Service, urging the IRS to revise Schedule H, Instructions to Acknowledge Housing-Health Link, April 1, 2015, http://www.aha.org/advocacy-issues/letter/2015/150401-aha-ltr-irs .pdf.

63. Sara Rosenbaum, Amber Rieke, and Maureen Byrnes, "Encouraging Nonprofit Hospitals to Invest in Community Building: The Role of IRS 'Safe Harbors,'" *Health Affairs Blog*, February 11, 2014, http://healthaffairs.org/blog/2014/02/11/ encouraging-nonprofit-hospitals-to-invest-in-community-building-the-role-of-irs -safe-harbors/.

64. U.S. Department of Treasury, "Additional Requirement for Charitable Hospitals," 79002.

65. This section is informed by the IRS responses to public comments to the 2012 Proposed Rules as well as the 2014 Final Rules in Department of Treasury, Internal Revenue Service, "Additional Requirement for Charitable Hospitals." See also Sara Rosenbaum, "Additional Requirements for Charitable Hospitals: Final Rules on Community Health Needs Assessments and Financial Assistance," *Health Affairs Blog*, January 23, 2015, http://healthaffairs.org/blog/2015/01/23/additional-requirements -for-charitable-hospitals-final-rules-on-community-health-needs-assessments-and -financial-assistance/.

66. U.S. Department of Treasury, "Additional Requirement for Charitable Hospitals," 78965.

67. Ibid., 79002.

68. Ibid., 78968.

69. Ibid., 79003–79004.

70. Beth Stephens, "Nonprofit Hospital Community Health Needs Assessments in Georgia," n.d., Atlanta: Georgia Watch Health Access Program, http://www.georgiawatch .org/wp-content/uploads/2015/06/Formatted-CHNA-Report-06022015-FINAL.pdf. Accessed July 31, 2015, accessed July 31, 2015.

71. Quoting Roland Labonte in Sana Loue, "Community Health Advocacy," *Journal of Epidemiology and Community Health* 60, no. 6 (June 2006): 458, doi:10.1136/jech.2004.023044. Here, I focus on community health advocacy groups that work to shape health care understandings, practices, and policy and not on the growing cadre of health or patient advocates who assist individual patients in negotiating the health care system.

72. Phil Brown and Stephen Zavestoski, "Social Movements in Health: An Introduction," *Sociology of Health and Illness* 26, no. 6 (September 2004): 679–694, doi:10.1111/j.0141–9889.2004.00413.x; Richard A. Couto, "Promoting Health at the Grass Roots," *Health Affairs* 9, no. 2 (May 1, 1990): 144–151, doi:10.1377/hlthaff.9.2.144; Steven Epstein, "Patient Groups and Health Movements," in *The Handbook of Science and Technology Studies*, ed. Edward J. Hackett et al., 3rd ed. (Cambridge, MA: MIT Press in cooperation with the Society for the Social Studies of Science, 2008), 499–539; Beatrix Hoffman et al., eds., *Patients as Policy Actors*, Critical Issues in Health and Medicine (New Brunswick, NJ: Rutgers University Press, 2011).

73. Charlie Eaton and Margaret Weir, "The Power of Coalitions: Advancing the Public in California's Public-Private Welfare State," *Politics and Society* 43, no. 1 (March 1, 2015): 3–32, doi:10.1177/0032329214558558.

74. Exceptions are found in Marcia Bayne-Smith, Yvonne Graham, and Sally Guttmacher, *Community-Based Health Organizations: Advocating for Improved Health*, 1st ed. (San Francisco: Jossey-Bass, 2005).

75. Epstein, "Patient Groups and Health Movements," 521.

76. Harper Jean Tobin, "The Next Phase of the Trans Movement," *Huffington Post*, June 13, 2014, http://www.huffingtonpost.com/harper-jean-tobin/the-next-phase-of-the-trans-movement_b_5475938.html. Emphasis in original.

77. Quoting Joe Dumit in Epstein, "Patient Groups and Health Movements," 510.

78. Roland Labonte, "Social Inclusion/Exclusion: Dancing the Dialectic," *Health Promotion International* 19, no. 1 (March 1, 2004): 117, doi:10.1093/heapro/dah112.

79. Iris Marion Young, "Activist Challenges to Deliberative Democracy," *Political Theory* 29, no. 5 (October 1, 2001): 670–690, doi:10.1177/0090591701029005004.

80. Bryan N. Massingale, *Racial Justice and the Catholic Church* (Maryknoll, NY: Orbis Books, 2010), 138.

81. National Latina Institute for Reproductive Health, "Texas," http://latinainstitute.org/en/texas, accessed September 6, 2015.

82. Forward Together, "Name Change FAQ," http://forwardtogether.org/about/name-change-faq, accessed September 6, 2015.

83. Labonte, "Social Inclusion/Exclusion," 120.

84. Cheryl A. Hyde, "Challenging Ourselves: Critical Self-Reflection on Power and Privilege," in *Community Organizing and Community Building for Health and Welfare*, ed. Meredith Minkler, 3rd ed. (New Brunswick, NJ: Rutgers University Press, 2012), 428–436.

85. Ibid.

86. Galen Ellis and Sheryl Walton, "Building Partnerships between Local Health Departments and Communities," in *Community Organizing and Community Building for Health and Welfare*, ed. Meredith Minkler, 3rd ed. (New Brunswick, NJ: Rutgers University Press, 2012), 131.

87. Angela Glover Blackwell and Raymond A. Colmenar, "Principles of Community Building: A Policy Perspective," in *Community Organizing and Community Building for Health and Welfare*, ed. Meredith Minkler, 3rd ed. (New Brunswick, NJ: Rutgers University Press, 2012), 423–427.

88. Maggie Potapchuk, "Paths Along the Way to Racial Justice: Four Foundation Case Studies," Philanthropic Initiative for Racial Equity Blog, *Critical Issues Forum*, 5 (June 18, 2014), 66, http://racialequity.org/docs/CIF5%20Casestudies.pdf.

89. Debra Strong et al., "Foundation's Consumer Advocacy Health Reform Initiative Strengthened Groups' Effectiveness," *Health Affairs* 30, no. 9 (September 1, 2011): 1799–1803, doi:10.1377/hlthaff.2011.0551.

90. Ibid., 1803.

91. Michelle C. Kegler et al., "Evaluation Findings on Community Participation in the California Healthy Cities and Communities Program," *Health Promotion International* 24, no. 4 (December 1, 2009): 307, doi:10.1093/heapro/dap036.

Conclusion

1. Robin Hawley Gorsline, quoting Ruth Frankenberg in "Shaking the Foundations: White Supremacy in the Theological Academy," in *Disrupting White Supremacy from Within: White People on What We Need to Do*, ed. Jennifer Harvey, Karin A. Case, and Robin Hawley Gorsline (Cleveland, OH: Pilgrim Press, 2004), 38.

Bibliography

Abelson, Julia, Erika Blacksher, Kathy Li, Sarah Boesveld, and Susan Goold. "Public Deliberation in Health Policy and Bioethics: Mapping an Emerging, Interdisciplinary Field." *Journal of Public Deliberation* 9, no. 1 (April 30, 2013). http://www.publicdeliberation.net/jpd/vol9/iss1/art5.

Abraido-Lanza, Anna F., Maria T. Chao, and Karen R. Florez. "Do Healthy Behaviors Decline with Greater Acculturation? Implications for the Latino Mortality Paradox." *Social Science and Medicine* 61, no. 6 (September 2005): 1243–1255. doi:10.1016/j.socscimed.2005.01.016.

Abrams, Lindsay. "Kind Neighbors Are Scarce, but Important." Survey conducted for the *Atlantic* in conjunction with GlaxoSmithKline. March 6, 2013. http://www.theatlantic.com/health/archive/2013/03/kind-neighbors-are-scarce-but-important/273375/.

"Advocates: Extending Medi-Cal to Undocumented Kids a First Step." *California Healthline*. July 7, 2015. http://californiahealthline.org/morning-breakout/advocates-extending-medical-to-undocumented-kids-a-good-first-step.

Aggleton, Peter, and Richard Parker. "Moving beyond Biomedicalization in the HIV Response: Implications for Community Involvement and Community Leadership among Men Who Have Sex with Men and Transgender People." *American Journal of Public Health* 105, no. 8 (August 2015): 1552–1558. doi:10.2105/AJPH.2015.302614.

Airhihenbuwa, Collins O. *Health and Culture: Beyond the Western Paradigm.* Thousand Oaks, CA: Sage, 1995.

Alvord, Lori Arviso, and Elizabeth Cohen. *The Scalpel and the Silver Bear.* New York: Bantam Books, 1999.

American Hospital Association. "Fast Facts on US Hospitals." 2014. http://www.aha.org/research/rc/stat-studies/fast-facts.shtml.

Anderson, Daren R., and J. Nwando Olayiwola. "Community Health Centers and the Patient-Centered Medical Home: Challenges and Opportunities to Reduce Health Care Disparities in America." *Journal of Health Care for the Poor and Underserved* 23, no. 3 (2012): 949–957.

Aronson, Louise. "Necessary Steps: How Health Care Fails Older Patients, and How It Can Be Done Better." *Health Affairs* 34, no. 3 (March 1, 2015): 528–532. doi:10.1377/hlthaff.2014.1238.

Baig, Arshiya A., Amanda Benitez, Cara A. Locklin, Amanda Campbell, Cynthia T. Schaefer, Loretta J. Heuer, Sang Mee Lee, et al. "Community Health Center Provider and Staff's Spanish Language Ability and Cultural Awareness." *Journal of Health Care for the Poor and Underserved* 25, no. 2 (2014): 527–545. doi:10.1353/hpu.2014.0086.

Barnes, Linda L. "Multiple Meanings of Chinese Healing in the United States." In *Religion and Healing in America*, edited by Linda L. Barnes and Susan Starr Sered, 307–331. Oxford and New York: Oxford University Press, 2005.

Barnes, Linda L., and Susan Starr Sered, eds. *Religion and Healing in America.* Oxford and New York: Oxford University Press, 2005.

Bayne-Smith, Marcia, Yvonne Graham, and Sally Guttmacher. *Community-Based Health*

Organizations: Advocating for Improved Health. 1st ed. San Francisco: Jossey-Bass, 2005.

Berkman, Lisa F., and Ichirō Kawachi. *Social Epidemiology.* New York: Oxford University Press, 2000.

Blacksher, Erika. "Participatory and Deliberative Practices in Health: Meanings, Distinctions, and Implications for Health Equity." *Journal of Public Deliberation* 9, no. 1 (April 30, 2013). http://www.publicdeliberation.net/jpd/vol9/iss1/art6.

Blacksher, Erika, Elizabeth Rigby, and Claire Espey. "Public Values, Health Inequality, and Alternative Notions of a 'Fair' Response." *Journal of Health Politics, Policy, and Law* 35, no. 6 (December 1, 2010): 889–920. doi:10.1215/03616878-2010-033.

Blackwell, Angela Glover, and Raymond A. Colmenar. "Principles of Community Building: A Policy Perspective." In *Community Organizing and Community Building for Health and Welfare*, edited by Meredith Minkler, 3rd ed., 423–427. New Brunswick, NJ: Rutgers University Press, 2012.

Bonham, Vence L., Toby Citrin, Stephen M. Modell, Tené Hamilton Franklin, Esther W. B. Bleicher, and Leonard M. Fleck. "Community-Based Dialogue: Engaging Communities of Color in the United States' Genetics Policy Conversation." *Journal of Health Politics, Policy, and Law* 34, no. 3 (June 1, 2009): 325–359. doi:10.1215/03616878–2009–009.

Boston University School of Medicine, Graduate Medical Sciences. "Our Roots: The Boston Healing Landscape Project." n.d. http://www.bumc.bu.edu/gms/maccp/about/our-roots-the-boston-healing-landscape-project. Accessed April 8, 2016.

Braveman, Paula, Susan Egerter, and David R. Williams. "The Social Determinants of Health: Coming of Age." *Annual Review of Public Health* 32, no. 1 (March 18, 2011): 381–398. doi:10.1146/annurev-publhealth-031210–101218.

Brennan, Virginia M. *Free Clinics: Local Responses to Health Care Needs.* Baltimore: Johns Hopkins University Press, 2013.

Brown, Phil, and Stephen Zavestoski. "Social Movements in Health: An Introduction." *Sociology of Health and Illness* 26, no. 6 (September 2004): 679–694. doi:10.1111/j.0141--9889.2004.00413.x.

Burge, Sandra K., and Teresa L. Albright. "Use of Complementary and Alternative Medicine among Family Practice Patients in South Texas." *American Journal of Public Health* 92, no. 10 (October 2002): 1614–1616.

Burton, Linda M., Susan P. Kemp, ManChui Leung, Stephen A. Matthews, and David T. Takeuchi, eds. *Communities, Neighborhoods, and Health: Expanding the Boundaries of Place.* Vol. 1: *Social Disparities in Health and Health Care.* New York and London: Springer, 2011.

Cahill, Lisa Sowle. *Theological Bioethics: Participation, Justice, and Change.* Moral Traditions Series. Washington, DC: Georgetown University Press, 2005.

Calabrese, Joseph D. *A Different Medicine: Postcolonial Healing in the Native American Church.* Oxford Ritual Studies. New York: Oxford University Press, 2013.

Callahan, Daniel. *What Kind of Life? The Limits of Medical Progress.* New York: Simon & Schuster, 1990.

Cassell, Eric J. *The Healer's Art: A New Approach to the Doctor-Patient Relationship.* Philadelphia: Lippincott, 1976.

Churchill, Larry R. "Toward a More Robust Autonomy: Revising the Belmont Report." In *Belmont Revisited: Ethical Principles for Research with Human Subjects*, edited by James F. Childress, Eric M. Meslin, and Harold T. Shapiro, 111–125. Washington, DC Georgetown University Press, 2005.

City of Huntington Park, California. "The Official Site of Huntington Park, CA!—

Commissions." http://www.hpca.gov/index.aspx?nid=60. Accessed August 12, 2015.

Cobb, John B., Jr. "Defining Normative Community." In *Rooted in the Land: Essays on Community and Place*, edited by William Vitek and Wes Jackson. New Haven, CT: Yale University Press, 1996.

Cohen, Barbara A. "Re: Designation of People with Serious Mental Illnesses as a Special Medically Underserved Population." Letter to Beth Rosenfeld, Health Resources and Services Administration, July 8, 2011. http://www.hrsa.gov/advisorycommittees/shortage/Meetings/20111012/publiccommenthorizonhouse.pdf.

"Community." *OED Online.* Oxford: Oxford University Press, March 2012.

Conrad, Peter. *The Medicalization of Society: On the Transformation of Human Conditions into Treatable Disorders.* Baltimore: Johns Hopkins University Press, 2007.

Corrigan, Janet M., and Elliott S. Fisher. "Accountable Health Communities: Insights from State Health Reform Initiatives." Lebanon, NH: Dartmouth Institute for Health Policy and Clinical Practice, November 2014. http://tdi.dartmouth.edu/research/evaluating/health-system-focus/accountable-care-organizations/accountable-health-communities:-insights-from-state-health-reform-initiatives.

Couto, Richard A. "Promoting Health at the Grass Roots." *Health Affairs* 9, no. 2 (May 1, 1990): 144–151. doi:10.1377/hlthaff.9.2.144.

Crawford O'Brien, Suzanne J., ed. *Religion and Healing in Native America: Pathways for Renewal.* Religion, Health, and Healing. Westport, CT: Praeger, 2008.

Cummins, Steven, Sarah Curtis, Ana V. Diez-Roux, and Sally Macintyre. "Understanding and Representing 'Place' in Health Research: A Relational Approach." *Social Science and Medicine*, special issue: "Placing Health in Context," 65, no. 9 (November 2007): 1825–1838. doi:10.1016/j.socscimed.2007.05.036.

Daniels, Norman. *Just Health: Meeting Health Needs Fairly.* Cambridge and New York: Cambridge University Press, 2008.

Dartmouth Medical School and Center for the Evaluative Clinical Sciences. *The Dartmouth Atlas of Health Care, 1996.* [Chicago]: AHA Press, 1996.

Davis, Karen, and Cathy Schoen. *Health and the War on Poverty: A Ten-Year Appraisal.* Washington, DC: Brookings Institution, 1978.

Dillon, Robin S. "Respect." In *The Stanford Encyclopedia of Philosophy*, edited by Edward N. Zalta, Spring 2014 ed. http://plato.stanford.edu/archives/spr2014/entries/respect.

———. "Respect and Care: Toward Moral Integration." *Canadian Journal of Philosophy* 22, no. 1 (March 1992): 105–132.

Eaton, Charlie, and Margaret Weir. "The Power of Coalitions: Advancing the Public in California's Public-Private Welfare State." *Politics and Society* 43, no. 1 (March 1, 2015): 3–32. doi:10.1177/0032329214558558.

Eckenwiler, Lisa A. *Long-Term Care and Globalization: An Ecological Approach.* Baltimore: Johns Hopkins University Press, 2012.

Eddy, Mary Baker. *Science and Health, with Key to the Scriptures.* Boston: First Church of Christ, Scientist, 1971.

Ellis, Galen, and Sheryl Walton. "Building Partnerships between Local Health Departments and Communities: Case Studies in Capacity Building and Cultural Humility." In *Community Organizing and Community Building for Health and Welfare*, edited by Meredith Minkler, 3rd ed., 131–147. New Brunswick, NJ: Rutgers University Press, 2012.

Emanuel, Ezekiel J. *The Ends of Human Life: Medical Ethics in a Liberal Polity.* Cambridge, MA: Harvard University Press, 1991.

Emanuel, Ezekiel J., and Charles Weijer. "Protecting Communities in Research: From a New Principle to Rational Protections." In *Belmont Revisited: Ethical Principles for Research with Human Subjects*, edited by James F. Childress, Eric M. Meslin, and Harold T. Shapiro, 165–183. Washington, DC: Georgetown University Press, 2005.

Epstein, Steven. "Patient Groups and Health Movements." In *The Handbook of Science and Technology Studies*, edited by Edward J. Hackett, Olga Amsterdamska, Michael Lynch, and Judy Wajcman, 3rd ed., 499–539. Cambridge, MA: MIT Press in cooperation with the Society for the Social Studies of Science, 2008.

Fadiman, Anne. *The Spirit Catches You and You Fall Down: A Hmong Child, Her American Doctors, and the Collision of Two Cultures*. 1st ed. New York: Farrar, Straus, & Giroux, 1997.

Fairchild, Patricia, and Pamela J. Byrnes. "Public Centers: A Discussion Monograph." Bethesda, MD: National Association of Community Health Centers, April 2014. http://www.nachc.com/client/documents/2014PublicCentersMonograph.pdf.

Farley, Margaret A. *Compassionate Respect: A Feminist Approach to Medical Ethics and Other Questions*. 2002 Madeleva Lecture in Spirituality. New York: Paulist Press, 2002.

———. "A Feminist Version of Respect for Persons." *Journal of Feminist Studies in Religion* 9, no. 1-2 (April 1, 1993): 183–198. doi:10.2307/25002208.

Fee, Elizabeth, and Nancy Krieger. "Understanding AIDS: Historical Interpretations and the Limits of Biomedical Individualism." *American Journal of Public Health* 83, no. 10 (October 1993): 1477–1486.

Fenway Institute, the Center for American Progress, Human Rights Campaign, and GLMA: Health Professionals Advancing LGBT, and Equality. "The Case for Designating LGBT People as a Medically Underserved Population and as a Health Professional Shortage Area Population Group." Boston: Fenway Institute, August 2014. http://fenwayhealth.org/documents/the-fenway-institute/policy-briefs/MUP_HPSA-Brief_v11-FINAL-081914.pdf.

Fleck, Leonard M. *Just Caring: Health Care Rationing and Democratic Deliberation*. Oxford and New York: Oxford University Press, 2009.

Fogarty, Colleen T. "Call It 'Jiffy Boob': What's Lacking When Care Has Assembly-Line Efficiency." *Health Affairs* 30, no. 11 (November 1, 2011): 2204–2207. doi:10.1377/hlthaff.2010.1106.

Folkemer, Donna C., Laura A. Spicer, Carl H. Mueller, Martha H. Somerville, Avery L. R. Brow, Charles Milligan, and Cynthia L. Boddie-Willis. "Hospital Community Benefits after the ACA: The Emerging Federal Framework." Hospital Community Benefits Program. Baltimore: Hilltop Institute, University of Maryland, Baltimore County, January 2011. https://folio.iupui.edu/handle/10244/1011.

Forward Together. "Name Change FAQ." http://forwardtogether.org/about/name-change-faq. Accessed September 6, 2015.

Fraser, Nancy. *Scales of Justice: Reimagining Political Space in a Globalizing World*. New Directions in Critical Theory. New York: Columbia University Press, 2009.

Frazer, Elizabeth, and Nicola Lacey. *The Politics of Community: A Feminist Critique of the Liberal-Communitarian Debate*. Toronto: University of Toronto Press, 1993.

Freidson, Eliot. *Profession of Medicine: A Study of the Sociology of Applied Knowledge*. New York: Harper & Row, 1970.

Friedman, Marilyn. "Feminism and Modern Friendship: Dislocating the Community." *Ethics* 99, no. 2 (January 1989): 275–290.

Galarneau, Charlene. "Health Care Sharing Ministries and Their Exemption from the Individual Mandate of the Affordable Care Act." *Journal of Bioethical Inquiry* 12, no. 2

(February 12, 2015): 269–282. doi:10.1007/s11673-015-9610-3.

———. "Nineteenth-Century Religious Hospitals: Community and Communities." Unpublished paper, April 1, 1991. Author's library.

———. "Still Missing: Undocumented Immigrants in Health Care Reform." *Journal of Health Care for the Poor and Underserved* 22, no. 2 (2011): 422–428. doi:10.1353/hpu.2011.0040.

Gawande, Atul. "The Cost Conundrum." *New Yorker*, June 1, 2009. http://www.newyorker.com/reporting/2009/06/01/090601fa_fact_gawande?printable=true&currentPage=all.

Geiger, H. Jack. "Community Health Centers: Health Care as an Instrument of Social Change." In *Reforming Medicine: Lessons of the Last Quarter Century*, edited by Victor W. Sidel and Ruth Sidel, 11–32. New York: Pantheon Books, 1984.

Gorsline, Robin Hawley. "Shaking the Foundations: White Supremacy in the Theological Academy." In *Disrupting White Supremacy from Within: White People on What We Need to Do*, edited by Jennifer Harvey, Karin A. Case, and Robin Hawley Gorsline, 33–62. Cleveland, OH: Pilgrim Press, 2004.

Gross, Michael L. "Speaking in One Voice or Many? The Language of Community." *Cambridge Quarterly of Healthcare Ethics* 13 (January 1, 2004): 28–33.

Harrison, Beverly Wildung. *Justice in the Making: Feminist Social Ethics*. Edited by Elizabeth M. Bounds, Pamela K. Brubaker, Jane E. Hicks, Marilyn J. Legge, Rebecca Todd Peters, and Traci C. West. Louisville, KY: Westminster John Knox Press, 2004.

Hatton, Melina Reid, and Lisa Gilden. Letter to Ms. Sunita Lough, Commissioner, Tax Exempt and Government Entities Division, Internal Revenue Service, urging the IRS to revise Schedule H, Instructions to Acknowledge Housing-Health Link, April 1, 2015. http://www.aha.org/advocacy-issues/letter/2015/150401-aha-ltr-irs.pdf.

Hehir, J. Bryan. "Social Justice." In *The HarperCollins Encyclopedia of Catholicism*, edited by Richard P. McBrien and Harold W. Attridge. San Francisco: HarperSanFrancisco, 1995.

Herman, Barbara. "The Scope of Moral Requirement." *Philosophy and Public Affairs* 30, no. 3 (Summer 2001): 227–256.

Hoffman, Beatrix Rebecca, Nancy Tomes, Rachel Grob, and Mark Schlesinger, eds. *Patients as Policy Actors*. Critical Issues in Health and Medicine. New Brunswick, NJ: Rutgers University Press, 2011.

Hollenbach, David. *Claims in Conflict: Retrieving and Renewing the Catholic Human Rights Tradition*. Woodstock Studies no. 4. New York: Paulist Press, 1979.

Holloway, Karla F. C. *Private Bodies, Public Texts: Race, Gender, and a Cultural Bioethics*. Durham, NC: Duke University Press, 2011.

Hutchinson, Tom A., ed. *Whole Person Care: A New Paradigm for the 21st Century*. New York: Springer, 2011.

Hyde, Cheryl A. "Challenging Ourselves: Critical Self-Reflection on Power and Privilege." In *Community Organizing and Community Building for Health and Welfare*, edited by Meredith Minkler, 3rd ed., 428–436. New Brunswick, NJ: Rutgers University Press, 2012.

Jewkes, Rachel, and Anne Murcott. "Meanings of Community." *Social Science and Medicine* 43, no. 4 (August 1996): 555–563. doi:10.1016/0277-9536(95)00439-4.

Kaptchuk, Ted J., and David M. Eisenberg. "Varieties of Healing. 1: Medical Pluralism in the United States." *Annals of Internal Medicine* 135, no. 3 (August 7, 2001): 189–195.

———. "Varieties of Healing. 2: A Taxonomy of Unconventional Healing Practices." *Annals of Internal Medicine* 135, no. 3 (August 7, 2001): 196–204.

Karpowitz, Christopher F., Tali Mendelberg, and Lee Shaker. "Gender Inequality in Deliberative Participation." *American Political Science Review* 106, no. 3 (August 2012): 533–547. doi:10.1017/S0003055412000329.

Kaslow, Nadine J., Annie M. Bollini, Benjamin Druss, Robert L. Glueckauf, Lewis R. Goldfrank, Kelly J. Kelleher, Annette Marie La Greca, et al. "Health Care for the Whole Person: Research Update." *Professional Psychology: Research and Practice* 38, no. 3 (2007): 278–289.

Kawachi, Ichiro. "The Relationship between Health Assets, Social Capital, and Cohesive Communities." In *Health Assets in a Global Context*, edited by Antony Morgan, Maggie Davies, and Erio Ziglio, 167–179. New York: Springer, 2010.

———. "Social Epidemiology." *Social Science and Medicine* 54, no. 12 (June 2002): 1739–1741. doi:10.1016/S0277-9536(01)00144-7.

Kegler, Michelle C., Julia Ellenberg Painter, Joan M. Twiss, Robert Aronson, and Barbara L. Norton. "Evaluation Findings on Community Participation in the California Healthy Cities and Communities Program." *Health Promotion International* 24, no. 4 (December 1, 2009): 300–310. doi:10.1093/heapro/dap036.

Kent, Edward. "Justice as Respect for Person." *Southern Journal of Philosophy* 6, no. 2 (1968): 70–77. doi:10.1111/j.2041-6962.1968.tb02028.x.

King, Patricia A. "Justice beyond Belmont." In *Belmont Revisited: Ethical Principles for Research with Human Subjects*, edited by James F. Childress, Eric M. Meslin, and Harold T. Shapiro, 136–147. Washington, DC: Georgetown University Press, 2005.

Labonte, Roland. "Social Inclusion/Exclusion: Dancing the Dialectic." *Health Promotion International* 19, no. 1 (March 1, 2004): 115–121. doi:10.1093/heapro/dah112.

Lawrence-Lightfoot, Sara. "Respect: On Witness and Justice." *American Journal of Orthopsychiatry* 82, no. 3 (July 2012): 447–454. doi:10.1111/j.1939-0025.2012.01174.x.

Leape, Lucian L., Miles F. Shore, Jules L. Dienstag, Robert J. Mayer, Susan Edgman-Levitan, S. Gregg, and Gerald B. Healy. "Perspective: A Culture of Respect, Part 1: The Nature and Causes of Disrespectful Behavior by Physicians." *Academic Medicine: Journal of the Association of American Medical Colleges* 87, no. 7 (July 2012): 845–852. doi:10.1097/ACM.0b013e318258338d.

Lebacqz, Karen. "We Sure Are Older But Are We Wiser?" In *Belmont Revisited: Ethical Principles for Research on Human Subjects*, edited by James F. Childress, Eric M. Meslin, and Harold T. Shapiro, 99–110. Washington, DC: Georgetown University Press, 2005.

Lefkowitz, Bonnie. *Community Health Centers: A Movement and the People Who Made It Happen*. Critical Issues in Health and Medicine. New Brunswick, NJ: Rutgers University Press, 2007.

Lin, Judy. "Sen. Ricardo Lara Drops Covered California Waiver for Immigrants." *Los Angeles Daily News*. September 4, 2015. http://www.dailynews.com/health/20150904/sen-ricardo-lara-drops-covered-california-waiver-for-immigrants.

Loue, Sana. "Community Health Advocacy." *Journal of Epidemiology and Community Health* 60, no. 6 (June 2006): 458–463. doi:10.1136/jech.2004.023044.

Loyd, Jenna. "Where Is Community Health? Racism, the Clinic, and the Biopolitical State." In *Rebirth of the Clinic: Places and Agents in Contemporary Health Care*, edited by Cindy Patton. Minneapolis: University of Minnesota Press, 2010.

MacQueen, Kathleen M., Eleanor McLellan, David S. Metzger, Susan Kegeles, Ronald P. Strauss, Roseanne Scotti, Lynn Blanchard, and Robert T. Trotter. "What Is Community? An Evidence-Based Definition for Participatory Public Health." *American Journal of Public Health* 91, no. 12 (December 2001): 1929–1938.

Marcus, Isabel. *Dollars for Reform: The OEO Neighborhood Health Centers.* Lexington, MA: Lexington Books, 1981.

Marshall, Wende Elizabeth. "Tasting Earth: Healing, Resistance Knowledge, and the Challenge to Dominion." *Anthropology and Humanism* 37, no. 1 (2012): 84–99. doi:10.1111/j.1548-1409.2012.01109.x.

Massingale, Bryan N. *Racial Justice and the Catholic Church.* Maryknoll, NY: Orbis Books, 2010.

Metzl, Jonathan M., and Helena Hansen. "Structural Competency: Theorizing a New Medical Engagement with Stigma and Inequality." *Social Science and Medicine,* special issue: "Structural Stigma and Population Health," 103 (February 2014): 126–133. doi:10.1016/j.socscimed.2013.06.032.

Mickey, Robert W. "Dr. StrangeRove; or, How Conservatives Learned to Stop Worrying and Love Community Health Centers." In *The Health Care Safety Net in a Post-reform World,* edited by Sara Rosenbaum and Mark A. Hall, 21–66. New Brunswick, NJ: Rutgers University Press, 2012.

Miles, Andrew. "Towards a *Medicine of the Whole Person*—Knowledge, Practice, and Holism in the Care of the Sick." *Journal of Evaluation in Clinical Practice,* special issue: "Evidence Based Medicine," 15, no. 6 (December 2009): 941–949.

Mishler, Elliot G. "Viewpoint: Critical Perspectives on the Biomedical Model." In *Social Contexts of Health, Illness, and Patient Care,* edited by Elliot G. Mishler, Lorna R. Amarasingham, Stuart T. Hauser, Samuel D. Osherson, Nancy E. Waxler, and Ramsay Liem, 1–23. New York: Cambridge University Press, 1981.

Mitchem, Stephanie Y., and Emilie Maureen Townes, eds. *Faith, Health, and Healing in African American Life.* Religion, Health, and Healing. Westport, CT, and London: Praeger, 2008.

Morehead, Mildred A. Book review of *The U.S. Experiment in Social Medicine: The Community Health Center Program, 1965–1986,* by Alice Sardell. *Journal of Public Health Policy* 10, no. 2 (Summer 1989): 266–267. doi:10.2307/3342687.

National Association of Community Health Centers. "Community Health Centers Past, Present, and Future: Building on 50 Years of Success." March 2015. http://www.nachc.com/client//PI_50th.pdf.

———. "Going beyond Primary Care: Health Centers Transform Health Care in Local Communities." 2013. https://www.nachc.com/client//Infographic_Final.pdf.

———. "Health Centers Addressing the Social Determinants of Health: Protocol for Responding to and Assessing Patient Assets, Risks, and Experiences (PRAPARE)." February 2015. https://www.nachc.com/client/PRAPARE%20abstract%20%20LC%20 overview%202%2026%2015.pdf.

———. "United States Health Center Fact Sheet, 2013." 2014. https://www.nachc.com/client//United_States_FS_2014.pdf.

National Immigration Law Center. "A Quick Guide to Immigrant Eligibility for ACA and Key Federal Means-Tested Programs, September 2015." *Access to Public Benefits—National Immigration Law Center.* https://www.nilc.org/wp-content/uploads/2015/11/imm-eligibility-quickguide-2015-09-21.pdf. Accessed April 2, 2016.

National Latina Institute for Reproductive Health. "Texas." http://latinainstitute.org/en/texas. Accessed September 6, 2015.

Nelson, Alondra. *Body and Soul: The Black Panther Party and the Fight against Medical Discrimination.* Minneapolis: University of Minnesota Press, 2011.

Nelson, Jennifer. *More than Medicine: A History of the Feminist Women's Health Movement.* New York: NYU Press, 2015.

Noble, Alice A., and Andrew L. Hyams. "Charitable Hospital Accountability: A Review and Analysis of Legal and Policy Initiatives." *Journal of Law, Medicine and Ethics* 26, no. 2 (Summer 1998): 116.

Payer, Lynn. *Medicine and Culture: Varieties of Treatment in the United States, England, West Germany, and France.* New York: Henry Holt, 1996.

Peal, Norma J., and Francisco A. R. Garcia. "Interdisciplinary Models for Women's Health: A Literature Review." *Archives: The International Journal of Medicine* 2, no. 1 (January 2009): 208–212.

Peel, Robert. *Health and Medicine in the Christian Science Tradition: Principle, Practice, and Challenge.* New York: Crossroad, 1988.

Potapchuk, Maggie. "Paths along the Way to Racial Justice: Four Foundation Case Studies." Philanthropic Initiative for Racial Equity Blog. *Critical Issues Forum* 5 (June 18, 2014). http://racialequity.org/docs/CIF5%20Casestudies.pdf.

Powers, Madison, and Ruth R. Faden. *Social Justice: The Moral Foundations of Public Health and Health Policy.* Issues in Biomedical Ethics. Oxford and New York: Oxford University Press, 2006.

Pradhan, Rachana. "California May Let Undocumented Immigrants Buy Obamacare." *POLITICO,* July 17, 2015. http://www.politico.com/story/2015/07/california-may-let-undocumented-immigrants-buy-obamacare-120249.

Proser, Michelle. "Deserving the Spotlight: Health Centers Provide High-Quality and Cost-Effective Care." *Journal of Ambulatory Care Management* 28, no. 4 (December 2005): 321–330.

Public Health and Welfare Act. 42 U.S.C. c. 6A(II)(D)(i): "Health Centers." 2015. Office of Law Revision Counsel: United States Code. http://uscode.house.gov/view.xhtml?path=/prelim@title42/chapter6A/subchapter2/partD/subpart1&edition=prelim.

Rasmussen, Larry L. *Moral Fragments and Moral Community: A Proposal for Church in Society.* Minneapolis: Fortress Press, 1993.

Rhoades, Everett R. *American Indian Health Innovations in Health Care, Promotion, and Policy.* Baltimore: Johns Hopkins University Press, 2000.

Rodriguez, Javier M., Arline T. Geronimus, John Bound, and Danny Dorling. "Black Lives Matter: Differential Mortality and the Racial Composition of the U.S. Electorate, 1970–2004." *Social Science and Medicine* 136/137 (July 2015): 193–199. doi:10.1016/j.socscimed.2015.04.014.

Rodwin, Marc A. "The Neglected Remedy: Strengthening Consumer Voice in Managed Care." *American Prospect* 34 (October 1997): 45–51.

Rosenbaum, Sara. "Additional Requirements for Charitable Hospitals: Final Rules on Community Health Needs Assessments and Financial Assistance." *Health Affairs Blog,* January 23, 2015. http://healthaffairs.org/blog/2015/01/23/additional-requirements-for-charitable-hospitals-final-rules-on-community-health-needs-assessments-and-financial-assistance/.

———. "Reinventing a Classic: Community Health Centers and the Newly Insured." In *The Health Care Safety Net in a Post-reform World,* edited by Mark A. Hall and Sara Rosenbaum, 67–90. New Brunswick, NJ: Rutgers University Press, 2012.

Rosenbaum, Sara, Amber Rieke, and Maureen Byrnes. "Encouraging Nonprofit Hospitals to Invest in Community Building: The Role of IRS 'Safe Harbors.'" *Health Affairs Blog.* February 11, 2014. http://healthaffairs.org/blog/2014/02/11/encouraging-nonprofit-hospitals-to-invest-in-community-building-the-role-of-irs-safe-harbors/.

Ruger, Jennifer Prah. *Health and Social Justice.* Oxford and New York: Oxford University Press, 2010.

Samuels, Michael E., and Sudha Xirasagar. "National Survey of Community Health Centers Board Chairs." Kansas City, MO: National Rural Health Association, May 2, 2005.

Sardell, Alice. *The U.S. Experiment in Social Medicine: The Community Health Center Program, 1965–1986.* Pittsburgh, PA: University of Pittsburgh Press, 1988.

Schlesinger, Mark. "Paradigms Lost: The Persisting Search for Community in U.S. Health Policy." *Journal of Health Politics, Policy, and Law* 22, no. 4 (August 1, 1997): 937–992. doi:10.1215/03616878-22-4-937.

Schlesinger, Mark, and Bradford Gray. "A Broader Vision for Managed Care, Part 1: Measuring the Benefit to Communities." *Health Affairs* 17, no. 3 (May 1, 1998): 152–168. doi:10.1377/hlthaff.17.3.152.

Schlesinger, Mark, Bradford Gray, Gerard Carrino, Mary Duncan, Michael Gusmano, Vincent Antonelli, and Jennifer Stuber. "A Broader Vision for Managed Care, Part 2: A Typology of Community Benefits." *Health Affairs* 17, no. 5 (September 1, 1998): 26–49. doi:10.1377/hlthaff.17.5.26.

Schoepflin, Rennie B. *Christian Science on Trial: Religious Healing in America.* Baltimore: Johns Hopkins University Press, 2002.

Scott, Robert A., Linda H. Aiken, David Mechanic, and Julius Moravcsik. "Organizational Aspects of Caring." *Milbank Quarterly* 73, no. 1 (January 1, 1995): 77–95. doi:10.2307/3350314.

Searcey, Dionne. "Hospitals Provide a Pulse in Struggling Rural Towns." Economy: A Shifting Middle. *New York Times*, April 29, 2015. http://www.nytimes.com/2015/04/30/business/economy/hospitals-provide-a-pulse-in-struggling-rural-towns.html.

Segall, Shlomi. *Health, Luck, and Justice.* Princeton, NJ: Princeton University Press, 2009.

Selznick, Philip. *The Moral Commonwealth: Social Theory and the Promise of Community.* Berkeley: University of California Press, 1992.

Shelley, Brian M., Andrew L. Sussman, Robert L. Williams, Alissa R. Segal, and Benjamin F. Crabtree. "'They Don't Ask Me So I Don't Tell Them': Patient-Clinician Communication about Traditional, Complementary, and Alternative Medicine." *Annals of Family Medicine* 7, no. 2 (April 3, 2009): 139–147. doi:10.1370/afm.947.

Sherwin, Susan. "A Relational Approach to Autonomy in Health Care." In *The Politics of Women's Health: Exploring Agency and Autonomy,* by the Feminist Health Care Ethics Research Network, coord. Susan Sherwin. Philadelphia: Temple University Press, 1998.

Shin, Peter, Jessica Sharac, and Sara Rosenbaum. "Community Health Centers and Medicaid at 50: An Enduring Relationship Essential for Health System Transformation." *Health Affairs* 34, no. 7 (July 1, 2015): 1096–1104. doi:10.1377/hlthaff.2015.0099.

Shortell, Stephen M., Pamela K. Washington, and Raymond J. Baxter. "The Contribution of Hospitals and Health Care Systems to Community Health." *Annual Review of Public Health* 30, no. 1 (April 2009): 373–383. doi:10.1146/annurev.publhealth.032008.112750.

Singh, Simone R., Gary J. Young, Shoou-Yih Daniel Lee, Paula H. Song, and Jeffrey A. Alexander. "Research and Practice: Analysis of Hospital Community Benefit Expenditures' Alignment with Community Health Needs: Evidence from a National Investigation of Tax-Exempt Hospitals." *American Journal of Public Health* 105, no. 5 (May 2015): 914–921. doi:10.2105/AJPH.2014.302436.

Smith, David M. *Geography and Social Justice.* Oxford and Cambridge, MA: Blackwell, 1994.

Starr, Paul. *The Social Transformation of American Medicine.* New York: Basic Books, 1982.

Stephens, Beth. "Nonprofit Hospital Community Health Needs Assessments in Georgia." n.d. Atlanta: Georgia Watch Health Access Program. http://www.georgiawatch .org/wp-content/uploads/2015/06/Formatted-CHNA-Report-06022015-FINAL.pdf. Accessed July 31, 2015.

Stone, John. "Race and Healthcare Disparities: Overcoming Vulnerability." *Theoretical Medicine and Bioethics* 23, no. 6 (November 2002): 499–518. doi:10.1023/A:1021524431845.

Strong, Debra, Debra Lipson, Todd Honeycutt, and Jung Kim. "Foundation's Consumer Advocacy Health Reform Initiative Strengthened Groups' Effectiveness." *Health Affairs* 30, no. 9 (September 1, 2011): 1799–1803. doi:10.1377/hlthaff.2011.0551.

"Tempers Flare as Huntington Park Appoints Undocumented Immigrants to City Commissions." CBS Los Angeles. August 4, 2015. http://losangeles.cbslocal.com/2015/08/04/ tempers-flare-when-huntington-park-appoints-2-undocumented-immigrants-to-city -commissions/.

Thompson, Juan. "'No Justice, No Respect': Why the Ferguson Riots Were Justified." *The Intercept.* December 1, 2014. https://firstlook.org/theintercept/2014/12/01/justice -respect-ferguson-riots-justified/.

Tobin, Harper Jean. "The Next Phase of the Trans Movement." *Huffington Post.* June 13, 2014. http://www.huffingtonpost.com/harper-jean-tobin/the-next-phase-of-the-trans -movement_b_5475938.html.

Tomes, Nancy. "Patients or Health-Care Consumers? Why the History of Contested Terms Matters." In *History and Health Policy in the United States: Putting the Past Back In,* edited by Rosemary A. Stevens, Charles E. Rosenberg, and Lawton R. Burns, 83–110. New Brunswick, NJ: Rutgers University Press, 2006.

Townes, Emilie Maureen. *Breaking the Fine Rain of Death: African American Health Issues and a Womanist Ethic of Care.* New York: Continuum, 1998.

———. *Womanist Ethics and the Cultural Production of Evil.* New York: Palgrave Macmillan, 2006.

U.S. Department of Health and Human Services, Health Resources and Services Administration. "Health Center Program Terminology Tip Sheet." n.d. bphc.hrsa.gov/ technicalassistance/healthcenterterminologysheet.pdf. Accessed July 11, 2015.

———. "Medically Underserved Areas/Populations: Guidelines for MUA and MUP Designation." June 1995. http://www.hrsa.gov/shortage/mua/index.html. Accessed May 24, 2015.

———. "Negotiated Rulemaking Committee on the Designation of Medically Underserved Populations and Health Professional Shortage Areas: Final Report to the Secretary" ("Final Report"). October 31, 2011. http://www.hrsa.gov/advisorycommittees/ shortage/nrmcfinalreport.pdf.

———. "2013 Health Center Data: National Program Grantee Data." Health Center Program. http://bphc.hrsa.gov/uds/datacenter.aspx. Accessed July 11, 2015.

U.S. Department of Health, Education, and Welfare, Office of the Secretary. *The Belmont Report: Ethical Principles and Guidelines for the Protection of Human Subjects of Research.* DHEW Publication nos. (OS) 78-0013 and 78-0014. Washington, DC: National Commission for the Protection of Human Subjects of Biomedical and Behavioral Research, April 18, 1979.

U.S. Department of Treasury, Internal Revenue Service. "Additional Requirement for Charitable Hospitals; Community Health Needs Assessments for Charitable Hospitals; Requirement of a Section 4959 Excise Tax Return and Time for Filing Return; Final Rule." *Federal Register* 79, no. 250 (December 31, 2014), 26 C.F.R. Parts 1, 53, and 602.

———. "Instructions for Schedule H (Form 990)." 2014.

Venkatapuram, Sridhar. *Health Justice: An Argument from the Capabilities Approach.* Cambridge: Polity, 2011.

Walzer, Michael. *Spheres of Justice: A Defense of Pluralism and Equality.* New York: Basic Books, 1983.

Williams, David R., Selina A. Mohammed, Jacinta Leavall, and Chiquita Collins. "Race, Socioeconomic Status, and Health: Complexities, Ongoing Challenges, and Research Opportunities." In *The Biology of Disadvantage: Socioeconomic Status and Health*, edited by Nancy E Adler and Judith Stewart. Boston: Blackwell, on behalf of the New York Academy of Sciences, 2010.

Wright, Brad. "Who Governs Federally Qualified Health Centers?" *Journal of Health Politics, Policy, and Law* 38, no. 1 (February 1, 2013): 27–55. doi:10.1215/03616878-1898794.

Wright, Brad, and Graham P. Martin. "Mission, Margin, and the Role of Consumer Governance in Decision Making at Community Health Centers." *Journal of Health Care for the Poor and Underserved* 25, no. 2 (2014): 930–947. doi:10.1353/hpu.2014.0107.

Young, Frank W., and Thomas A. Lyson. "Structural Pluralism and All-Cause Mortality." *American Journal of Public Health* 91, no. 1 (January 2001): 136–138.

Young, Iris Marion. "Activist Challenges to Deliberative Democracy." *Political Theory* 29, no. 5 (October 1, 2001): 670–690. doi:10.1177/0090591701029005004.

———. "Asymmetrical Reciprocity: On Moral Respect, Wonder, and Enlarged Thought." In *Intersecting Voices: Dilemmas of Gender, Political Philosophy, and Policy*, 38–59. Princeton, NJ: Princeton University Press, 1997.

———. "Gender as Seriality: Thinking about Gender as a Social Collective." In *Intersecting Voices: Dilemmas of Gender, Political Philosophy, and Policy*, 12–37. Princeton, NJ: Princeton University Press, 1997.

———. *Justice and the Politics of Difference.* Princeton, NJ: Princeton University Press, 1990.

Zuckerman, David. "Hospitals Building Healthier Communities: Embracing the Anchor Mission." Takoma Park, MD: Democracy Collaborative at the University of Maryland, March 2013. http://community-wealth.org/sites/clone.community-wealth.org/files/downloads/Zuckerman-HBHC-2013.pdf.

Index

ACA. *See* Patient Protection and Affordable Care Act (ACA, 2010)

accessibility, 14

advocacy groups. *See* community health advocacy groups

African Americans, 13, 17, 24, 85, 115n73

Airhihenbuwa, Collins O., 12–13, 106n22

Alvord, Lori Arviso, 14–15

Aronson, Louise, 69

The Belmont Report: Ethical Principles and Guidelines for the Protection of Human Subjects of Research (National Commission for the Protection of Human Subjects of Biomedical and Behavioral Research), 57

Belmont Revisited (commentaries on *Belmont Report*), 57, 58

bioethics, 37, 56–57, 116n83

biomedical community, 11–13, 18, 29, 43, 69, 70

blood transfusions, 14, 29

Boston Healing Landscape Project, 13

Boston Women's Health Book Collective, 94

Brown, Jerry, 67

Burton, Linda M., 16

Bush, George W., 83

Cahill, Lisa Sowle, 71

California, 67, 95, 97–98

The California Endowment (TCE), 95, 97–98

Callahan, Daniel, 16–17, 67

capabilities approaches to health care justice, 32–38; Powers and Faden on, 32, 35–36, 36–37, 110n58; Ruger on, 32–34, 35, 37; Venkatapuram on, 32, 34–35. *See also* liberal theories of health care justice

care, definition, 16–17

care respect, 58

care work, 19, 69

Cassell, Eric, 68

Catholic Church, 18, 71–72

Center for the Evaluative Clinical Sciences (Dartmouth), 12

charity care, 90

CHCs. *See* community health centers (CHCs)

Child Health Insurance Program, 66

Chinese medicine, 13

CHNAs. *See* community health needs assessments (CHNAs)

Christian Science, 13

chronically ill persons, 75

Churchill, Larry, 57

citizens, definition, 41

Cobb, John, 9

community: definition, 3, 8–11; geographic, 63–67, 76–77

community benefits, 4, 11, 19–21; CHNA requirements, 90–91, 92

community good, health care as, 7–21

community health advocacy groups, 5, 80, 94–98, 99, 121n71; condition-based, 19; effective voice/just participation, 96–98, 102; geographic inclusivity, 100; support for, 94–95; whole-person care, 95–96

community health centers (CHCs), 3, 5, 17–18, 80–89, 98, 101; early history of, 80–82; effective voice, 84, 87–89, 102; federal funding policy, 80, 82, 83–86, 84–86; geographic inclusivity, 84, 89, 99; legislation authorizing, 82, 88; private nonprofits vs. public centers, 88–89; services offered by, 86, 89; terminology relating to, 82–83, 117n15; whole-person care, 84, 86–87

community health needs assessments (CHNAs), 5, 80, 89–94, 98, 99; addressing needs identified by, 93; community-benefits requirements in, 90–91, 92; early history of, 89–90; effective voice, 92–94, 101–102; geographic inclusivity, 91; tax policy, 89–93, 99, 100, 101, 121n62; whole-person care, 92–93

About the Author

Charlene Galarneau is assistant professor of Women's and Gender Studies at Wellesley College. She received a doctorate in religion from Harvard University with a concentration in religious social ethics and health policy and holds master's degrees from Harvard University and the Iliff School of Theology (Denver). Her academic endeavors are inspired by her early work with rural community/migrant health centers and the communities they serve.

Galarneau's research focuses on the ethics of health care and public health, and feminist bioethics. Her work appears in the *Journal of Bioethical Inquiry*, *Health and Human Rights*, the *Hastings Center Report*, the *American Journal of Bioethics*, *Public Health Ethics*, and the *Journal of Health Care for the Poor and Underserved*.

Available titles in the Critical Issues in Health and Medicine series:

Matthew Smith, *An Alternative History of Hyperactivity: Food Additives and the Feingold Diet*

Rosemary A. Stevens, Charles E. Rosenberg, and Lawton R. Burns, eds., *History and Health Policy in the United States: Putting the Past Back In*

Barbra Mann Wall, *American Catholic Hospitals: A Century of Changing Markets and Missions*

Frances Ward, *The Door of Last Resort: Memoirs of a Nurse Practitioner*

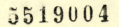